The Power of
the Streak

A Clear Path to Consistent Exercise and Staying Motivated Over Time

KARA WOOD

DEDICATION

To Tyler, M, and T:
My Everyday Inspiration;
And to the Judge and Bethany:
My Streak Inspiration

ACKNOWLEDGMENTS

The list of people who have helped and encouraged me through the process of writing this book is so very long. Thank you to my husband, parents, mother-in-law, brother, and sisters, who all believe in me to a fault. Thank you to my dear friends and family members who took precious time to read drafts and help me work through countless and often ridiculous ideas. Thank you to the Judge, whose mentoring and encouragement know no bounds.

Thank you to Joanna Penn, Johnny B. Truant, and Sean Platt, whose books showed me that this writing/publishing thing was possible.

Thank you to Lizbe Coetzee for her beautiful and artistic cover design.

Finally, thank you to my editor, Dianne Giambusso, for her thoughtful suggestions.

CONTENTS

PART ONE: THE STREAK CONCEPT

1 INTRODUCTION 3

2 WHY A STREAK? 11

3 TOO MUCH PRESSURE? 23

PART TWO: STARTING A STREAK

4 DEFINE YOUR EXERCISE REQUIREMENT 31

5 SET YOUR MINIMUM MILEAGE, LAPS, OR TIME 59

6 SET YOUR MINIMUM DAYS PER WEEK 65

7 SET YOUR TARGET WORKOUT TIME OF DAY 69

PART THREE: MAINTAINING THE STREAK

8 RECORD YOUR PROGRESS 77

9 PLAN FOR THE WEEK AHEAD 82

10 SACRIFICE WHEN NECESSARY 85

11 SETBACKS AND INJURIES 92

PART FOUR: BEYOND THE STREAK

12 SET OTHER FITNESS GOALS TO ACHIEVE
WHILE KEEPING UP YOUR STREAK 99

13 STREAKING IN AREAS OTHER THAN FITNESS 106

14 INSPIRING OTHERS THROUGH YOUR FITNESS
STREAK 109

PART ONE:

THE STREAK CONCEPT

1 INTRODUCTION

I'm an ordinary person. A wife and mom of two with a demanding full-time job and a particularly cynical view of the world. I'm in my late thirties, live in suburbia, and spend about two-and-a-half hours per day driving kids to school and myself to work and back. I've never been a standout athlete. Well into adulthood, I had zero interest in fitness or working out. But one day, Memorial Day of 2010 to be exact, I reluctantly decided to give running a shot.

Why running? I needed some cardio: stat. An unfortunate capture of me wearing a not-so-flattering dress at my sister's wedding finally gave me the push needed to get off the couch and take up an activity that might actually help my organs. But again, why running? Truth is, I was lazy and it seemed easy. You put on some shoes and you go. No worrying about joining a gym, dealing with gawkers, buying expensive equipment, or learning something new.

The goal seemed simple enough: run five days a week, every week, for at least a mile. Although simplistic in theory, the impact is lasting. Fast forward twelve years later, and I haven't missed a single week. *Not one.* For more than 600 weeks in a row, I've run through the chaos of everyday life, through two pregnancies and childbirths, through countless vacations, injuries, and setbacks. How? The Power of the Streak.

I know what you're thinking (or at least I'd be thinking it). "She's clearly a nut. One of those obsessive and/or preachy types. And she's probably a liar to boot."

I'm here to tell you, sure, my mental stability may have been questioned from time to time, but that has nothing to do with the streak. (Did I mention I have kids?) And no, I'm not preachy about the Power of the Streak. In fact, most people who know me don't even know or care about my streak. If someone hears about it and shows interest, I'll tell them what they want to know, but I'm not going to beg anyone to listen to me talk about it. I'm not obsessive either, except when it comes to my coffee habit. As for my integrity about the streak situation, my husband can attest to all the strange things I've done over the years to keep the streak alive. But only to keep the streak alive. Otherwise, I'm totally normal. I swear.

So, why would I write this book? Well, completing a book has always been one of those life goals— something I've wanted to do but I've never had the drive to finish. I've had incomplete books lying around the house for ages and countless ideas of book topics.

Then I heard somewhere that the most effective books are those that can actually change human behavior. At first, I thought nothing of the statement. But then it dawned on me (during a run, of course) that my behavior and, eventually my life, changed in a *HUGE* way by simply deciding to start a running streak all those years ago. And it really wasn't hard to do.

This realization jump-started my motivation to write. If I can help others start—and maintain—their own fitness streaks by explaining all the ins and outs, then the effort of writing it all down will be more than worth it. Plus, I'll actually accomplish my book goal! Bonus!

Let's start with my streak inspiration. In late 2007, I graduated from law school and immediately went to work as a staff lawyer at a courthouse. Those college and law school years had taken their toll on the ol' physique, but I was in denial. I had been tall and slender through high school and most of college without having to do much exercise. My metabolism would get me through the rest of my life, too!

My boss for the post-law school job, who remains my boss today, is an unapologetic fitness fanatic. The kind who can simultaneously be inspiring and irritating to a twenty-something. On one of my first days, while handing me a file that was so large I couldn't see over it, he told me the reason why he worked out every day for at least thirty minutes: because the President did it. He declared, "If the President can find time to do it, so can I." I politely smiled, nodded my head, silently judged, and attempted to find my way back to my office to figure out how to be a lawyer.

But the story stuck with me. I found myself wondering: "Does he really work out Every. Single. Day? Does the President? Ludicrous!" My boss, just before landing a judgeship, had been a federal prosecutor in charge of a district with hundreds of employees and spanning most of the state of Florida.

In addition to being in charge, he traveled regularly between different offices and often tried cases. He didn't seem like the kind of guy who had a lot of free time on his hands.

As if he sensed my doubt about the every-day workout, my boss would not-so-subtly tell me each morning how he woke up at 5:00 a.m., 5:30 a.m., insert any other insane time, just to get in his thirty minutes. He'd be frustratingly energetic. Ugh, morning people. And sometimes he'd go running or biking after work as well! How was this happening? And why did I need to witness it?

My boss pushed me for more than two years to start a fitness routine to no avail. He pulled out all the stops, including placing in my office chair countless workout ideas, fitness articles, and suggestions on equipment to try. But I was newly married, possibly immature, trying to find my way in my career, and way more interested in libations than fitness. (I'm sure none of this remains true.) Plus, it was fun to rebel where I could. I *refused* to be someone's passion project!

Then came the dress picture. In the spring of 2010, my younger sister got married in a beautiful ceremony on the river. All of the bridesmaids—myself included—wore strapless, cobalt blue knee-length gowns that perfectly complimented the shades of the water and the gorgeous hydrangea bouquets. A real dream wedding.

A few weeks later, I was sitting at work trying to figure out what "substantial evidence" meant when, ding, an email came through with the wedding pictures. Yay! A fun distraction! While on my lunch break (go with it), I clicked the link, excited to check out the surely-stunning pics. My sister looked naturally and effortlessly beautiful. I'm talking Princess-Kate-on-a-barely-breezy-day kind of beautiful. Her adoring husband was nothing short of dapper in his tux. These were some great photos.

Next came the wedding party. *Gasp.* "Is that ME? Do I really look like that? What's with all the extra . . ." Mortified, I quickly clicked the "x" and then tried to convince myself it wasn't that bad.

Now, those of you who have had one of these experiences know exactly what I'm talking about. Go ahead. Describe the picture out loud. You'll feel better.

Those of you who haven't had one of these experiences are either perfect, in denial, or have an advanced degree in photogenics.

Whether or not you've experienced photo realism in the way I did, there's a reason you picked up this book. I'm here to help, not judge. The reality is, I wasn't particularly large in the photo. Maybe some wouldn't even notice the extra baggage and overly-aggressive push-up bra combined with strangely broad shoulders (yes, you remembered correctly, the dress was strapless—a brutal combo). But I had gotten to a point of being uncomfortable with the way I looked and felt. I couldn't rely on my metabolism anymore. Something had to give.

I let things simmer. I threatened to start exercising. I even thought about joining a gym. But it wasn't until Memorial Day weekend of 2010 that I took real action.

Within weeks of the wedding picture realization, my two sisters and I took our mother to Savannah, Georgia for the long holiday weekend. Savannah is a delightful place for a "girls' trip" because of its old architecture, great food, and charming people. The city's unofficial slogan—at least according to multiple t-shirts and storefronts—is: "Treats and memories made from scratch."

One morning, we were to wake up at the crack of dawn to stand in line for breakfast at a particularly popular no-reservation-taking restaurant. Waking up early? Not my thing. Standing in line, slightly hungover, in the morning? Not my thing. But you do these things on trips with people you love.

On the designated morning, I heard the alarm go off. Despite wanting to scream, I managed to keep it in. When I rolled over, I noticed that my trusty sister/roommate/drinking pal had gone missing. Where was she? Still groggy, I asked my mom if she knew. It turns out my sister was *running*. What?!

I mean, it was no secret that this sister was into fitness and working out and all the healthy things. But she had just spent a fun night out drinking with us, we were getting up early to go stand in some line, and she had the self-motivation to get up even earlier to go for a run? On vacation?

I tried to be disgusted, but it was hard. Here I was, unsatisfied with how I looked and felt, but not doing a darn thing about it. Yet, here was my sister, disciplined enough to know she needed to run and doing it at the crack of dawn, post-night-out.

We stood in line, ate the breakfast, and drove home. After I threw my overnight bag in the doorway ("I'll unpack later…"), I dug a pair of old tennis shoes out of my closet, put them on, and committed to running a minimum of a mile, five days a week, every week. Just like that.

As I proclaimed this commitment to my confused husband while walking out the door, he just stared at me and said, "Okay, be careful," as he probably chalked it up to another one of my phases. Little did he know, he'd be telling me to be careful as I walked out the door 3,000 more times *and counting*. And he surely didn't realize that years down the road, he'd start his own exercise streak. More on this later.

Beyond my running streak, I've completed handfuls of organized runs and even two half marathons: one trailing my sister (well, she did a full marathon, naturally) and one trailing my boss. A sort of ironic tribute to my great inspirations.

The real takeaway here is this: the Power of the Streak can exist in all of us, even those of us who are not particularly interested in fitness or exercise. All it takes is commitment, clear parameters, drive, and focus.

In this book, you'll first learn the benefits of a streak. I'll show you how having a streak does not add pressure to your life, no matter your circumstance. We'll discuss several different exercise ideas for a streak—it most definitely doesn't have to be running—and how to set your minimum exercise requirement. We'll talk about having a target time of day to work out but also being flexible when necessary. We'll tackle how to decide whether to have a daily streak or a days-per-week streak. Also, we'll discuss maintaining the streak, including tracking your progress, planning for the week ahead, and dealing with setbacks and injuries. Finally, we'll talk about inspiration beyond your streak in the form of ways to push yourself with more exercise, streaks in other areas of life, and inspiring others with your workout streak.

Throughout the book, I often draw on my own experience and the experiences of those in my close circle who have their own exercise streaks. The stories are powerful because they show how a commitment and clear parameters translate to long-lasting exercise success, even in those who have struggled mightily in the past with routinized exercise. The bottom line is that the Power of the Streak can exist in all of us—even a cynic like me.

2 WHY A STREAK?

We are all familiar with the concept of a streak in some form. If you're a sports fan, you can spout off how many games in a row your team has won or lost. Or maybe you can rattle off the number of games in a row that Joe DiMaggio got a hit in 1941. If you're a parent, you can recall off the top of your head how many times you've made it through the dreaded morning school drop-off line before the first bell rings. (Three and counting . . .) If you're in business, you probably know the last time your company had a negative quarter, or rather, how many consecutive positive quarters the company has had. Whether you realize it or not, streaks exist—only to be broken—everywhere.

So how does this streak idea apply to fitness? The skeptic should rightly ask at this point, "Why should I buy into this potentially ridiculous idea of a workout streak?" I asked that question for two and a half years before buying in. As usual, I was slow on the uptake. Once I finally acquiesced, the benefits became clear.

The answer to the question is three-fold. First, the workout streak ensures discipline in an area of your life where it is most likely lacking. Second, it forces accountability to yourself. Third, and far most important, keeping the streak alive means *keeping the workout going.*

2.1 The Streak Ensures Discipline

The first major benefit of a workout streak is that it ensures discipline. Let's face it: if you picked up this book you likely have a major lack of discipline in the area of fitness. Maybe you don't currently work out at all. Maybe you "try" to work out a certain number of times per week. But then those happy hours or soccer practices or PFA meetings get in the way, and before you know it, another week has passed without meeting your workout goal. Maybe you do work out regularly, but you've never considered or tried a workout streak.

Think of the area in your life where you have the most discipline. Is it work? Housework? Yard work? Something else? What makes you so disciplined in that area?

If it's work, maybe your stellar discipline comes from the simple reality that you have to show up and be productive or face the axe. Maybe you actually enjoy your job. Maybe your parents instilled a strong work ethic in you. Maybe you're vying for a promotion or a raise. Whatever the reason, whatever the motivation, you have either consciously or subconsciously prioritized your job and you've taken steps to ensure that you stay disciplined in performing it.

What about housework or yard work? Are you one of those people who has spotless floors, glimmering cabinets, and the whole family's laundry done every

Sunday night? Does your front lawn look like a perfect green carpet from a self-mowing job completed every week without fail? Do you water the lawn like clockwork every day your city allows (and maybe an extra snuck in here or there)? If any of this describes you, I simply cannot relate.

In all seriousness, though, why are you rabid about the housework or the yard work? What makes you disciplined enough to ensure it all gets done? I'll tell you. You've decided that the housework or yard work is important to you, and you've prioritized it.

What if you could prioritize discipline in the area of fitness without even really having to think or worry about it? With a streak, exercise moves up on your priority list in the same way that a nakedly-ambitious person works a room full of influencers: swiftly, flawlessly, and with ease. Even better, the dreaded exercise transforms into an essential and welcome part of your day. That is the Power of the Streak.

A streak is one of the easier lifestyle changes you can make: once you commit to doing it and set the parameters, the rest falls into place. *It's something you know you have to do.* A streak even makes it easier for your spouse, boyfriend or girlfriend, family, or close friends to understand your need—not desire—to work out on a regular basis. In other words, it makes for easier support in your lifestyle change. If you communicate your streak and its importance, it will become accepted as an essential part of your day, no matter how busy life may be.

My "streak week" starts on Monday. Depending on how busy the week has been, by Friday I may have run all five required days or maybe I've only had time for three. How many runs I've completed during the week dictates how many times I have to run over the weekend. The famous phrase in my household to start each weekend is, "Do you have to run both days?" The way this question is posed by my husband shows his complete acceptance that the streak must stay alive, his willingness to help out with doing what needs to be done for it to stay alive, and even planning ahead! *Whaaa?!*

2.2 The Streak Forces Self-Accountability

The second major benefit of a workout streak is forced self-accountability. How many times have you told yourself this week that you'll go to the gym or get on the exercise bike? How many times have you kept your word? Even if you've met your workout goals this week (yay!), chances are you have difficulty maintaining them for any real length of time.

When you actually make it to the gym, are you really working out like you told yourself you would? Or is it more of a spectator sport? When you get on the bike, do you stay on as long as you had originally intended? Do you do ten miles as you said you would, or stop at five because you're over it?

The streak eliminates the opportunity to cheat on yourself in your workout routine. It forces you to be accountable to yourself. You know exactly what you have to do to keep the streak alive, and you know how many days per week you have to do it. There is no room for excuses or fudging the numbers. You either do what you need to do or the streak is broken.

Self-accountability is no easy feat, especially if it's in an area of life where you struggle. For this reason, the concept of being accountable to someone other than yourself when you want to meet a goal, including fitness, has become increasingly popular. A few ways to accomplish this include accountability groups, accountability buddies, and focused classes.

Accountability groups are not new conceptually but seem to be popping up lately as rapidly as mask sellers in 2020. The basic idea behind an accountability group is that people come together to discuss their progress and challenges in meeting particular goals. A sort of "safe place" where ideas can flow freely and others can tell you what you're doing right and wrong.

There are multitudes of accountability groups in existence. A quick internet search will reveal accountability groups for fitness, dieting, religion, job seeking, addiction, financial goals, and so on.

Some accountability groups are effective, some not so much. When effective, these groups provide motivation and comfort, unite people in a common cause, and actually hold members accountable to each other in their goal setting. Common reasons for failure or ineffectiveness for the group concept include inconsistency in attendance, members having an "enabling" attitude, personalities not "meshing," and inauthenticity. Plus, if you already lead a busy life, it can be hard to set aside a couple of hours on a weeknight to drive to and attend one of these group meetings on top of setting aside the needed time to workout.

An accountability buddy is someone you know and trust who you assign to hold you accountable to what you say you're going to do. This person can be going through the same journey as you or not. For instance, I could ask my bestie to meet me at the gym twice a week, or I could ask her to simply check to see if I've gone to the gym.

This idea, like accountability groups, can be effective or ineffective. First, it can be difficult to find a person you know and trust with the same goals you have or who is willing to hold you accountable. Second, the person has to be reliable or you'll be set up for failure. Even if your girlfriend says she will meet you at the gym twice a week, if she is not particularly reliable, it will do you no good. If you show up to the gym at your scheduled rendezvous time only to be met with a text that says, "So sorry, I'm stuck at work. Have fun without me!" it's frustrating and demoralizing. Third, depending on your accountability buddy's personality and motivation, it could be easy to talk her into going out for a drink rather than going to the gym. Or, if she's only supposed to be checking to see if you went to the gym, if you give her your excuse about why you didn't, she could easily accept it and let you off the hook.

An organized exercise class is another form of being accountable to someone other than yourself. Typically offered by a gym or fitness-related business, these classes have varied in popularity over time. Individuals signing up for the classes usually pay a fee to attend. Different types of classes are offered depending on your fitness level and your exercise interest, and the classes are run by an expert in that area. A few examples are spinning classes, Orangetheory, and boot-camp style classes (think of the people in parks or under bridges or in mall parking lots being yelled at by a very fit-looking man or woman with a boom box microphone).

Organized classes have their pros and cons. On the pro side, an organized class is typically a great workout. You are likely to learn new moves and ensure you're doing them with the right technique. Also, something about working out in front of others doing the same motivates people to work harder. Once more, knowing the specific day and time of your class can help you prioritize getting there.

On the con side, the classes can be expensive. The set times lead to some inflexibility in when you can go. The idea of working out in front of people might make you squirm. Also problematic: you have to actually show up to the class to be held accountable in any way. It's not likely that your spin instructor is going to call and ask you why you didn't do the 10:00 a.m. ride like you thought you would.

A workout streak is unique from an accountability perspective because it does not require anyone else to hold you accountable, but at the same time, it ensures self-accountability. It's almost like the streak is your accountability buddy. But the streak won't leave you stranded at the gym or be talked into going to happy hour instead of working out. Your streak is as reliable as they come. If you break the streak for a meaningless reason, you know it's over. You've let yourself, and your streak, down. That is some powerful accountability.

2.3 The Streak Keeps the Workout Going

The most obvious and most impactful benefit of a workout streak is that it keeps you working out. It truly changes your behavior. This isn't the latest fad or designer diet or way to save money by skipping your daily latte (good luck with that). The streak, by definition, means you will keep working out indefinitely. It's the closest thing you'll find to a "magic pill" that will get you in shape.

Why do you keep trying to exercise even after you fail? Why does anyone keep trying? Because next time could be your time; the time that something clicks. The Power of the Streak is truly different than these other times you've tried. It's not about generally committing to exercise or committing to getting in shape. It's about committing to a streak: an indefinite period of time that you'll keep your exercise going.

Why did I commit that Memorial Day to running a minimum of a mile for five days a week, every single week? Because I know myself. I know that if I had said, "I'm going to start running," or "I'll try to run five days a week," or anything that would give me the slightest wiggle room, I would be back on the couch, indefinitely, within a couple weeks at most. But with clear commitment and clear parameters, it became easy to implement. Before I knew it, a year had passed. Then five. Then ten. And it doesn't even feel hard. Seriously.

My husband, Tyler, is the strongest example of the Power of the Streak to keep someone working out. Unlike me, Tyler was a standout athlete. He even landed a scholarship to play basketball in college. But during college, he badly injured his back, and he'd eventually require significant surgery during the first year of our marriage.

We've all heard horror stories about back injuries and surgeries. While I wouldn't describe Tyler's post-surgical situation as a horror story per se, his back pain remains a daily challenge even fourteen years later.

Even though he struggles mightily with the pain, Tyler has always wanted to fight through it to maintain some level of athleticism and fitness. But he never had any workout routine catch on for any significant length of time. For years, this led to a sort of roller coaster pattern of him latching onto some workout fad, losing forty pounds, only to fall off the wagon within months and put all the weight back on. Then the next year, he'd try something else and the cycle would continue.

There was the pick-up basketball phase. This phase led to a trip to the emergency room and my subsequent banning of basketball at the local pick-up spot. (He has a special souvenir scar on his head that we affectionately refer to as "Eloh," or "Hole" spelled backwards.) There was the "Insanity" phase. (Oh, how I don't miss the workout DVDs randomly spread throughout the house.) This workout fad was almost literally insane: too hard on his body and not sustainable. There was the gym elliptical phase. This machine was good for less impact on his back but proved difficult to maintain for any significant period because it was still quite painful.

All of a sudden, about six years into our marriage, I noticed that the cycle had come to a complete halt. He wasn't even trying new things anymore. He was frustrated by his limitations and the lack of sustainability in the things he had tried. He was deflated.

He remained deflated for years.

Then, in June 2019, more than a decade after the roller coaster cycle had started, Tyler decided to give the streak a try. I never really pushed the streak idea for him because of his limitations, but he had seen me doing it for years and he became intrigued. What exercise would be sustainable indefinitely, though, for a guy who has serious back problems?

Tyler's streak idea came to him while taking our little girl to the local club pool to teach her how to swim. He'd swim laps for his streak. He had been a swimmer in high school, so he was comfortable in the water. It was low in impact but high in cardio. Perfect.

So starting in June 2019, Tyler committed to swimming twenty laps per day, five days a week. And it stuck.

His story is so powerful because he tried, and failed, to keep up a workout routine for more than a decade before committing to a workout streak. Once he committed and set clear parameters, the rest fell into place. He's faced some serious challenges keeping a swimming streak alive, but he's done it now for more than three years and counting. There is something different about a streak.

Another inspiring example of the Power of the Streak to keep the workout going is my friend, Megan. We work together. Megan ran some in her late twenties and into her thirties, but then life got in the way. By the time I met her, she had a husband, young twin daughters and an older stepdaughter, and had just started a new, challenging job. She also had a lingering issue with some muscles in her foot that made it difficult and frustrating to exercise.

When Megan first joined our team, she often heard my boss and me talking about our weekend runs. She would see us go out after work for a run before heading home. My boss, always the motivator, started encouraging her to try some sort of regular exercise routine.

Megan explains that she had never thought of the concept of a workout streak until she saw what we were doing. She was particularly moved by the fact that my boss and I pushed through no matter how busy our day had been, no matter what was going on in our lives, and no matter how we felt.

Megan decided to try her own streak. She liked the idea because she viewed it as a unique challenge, almost like she could be in competition with herself. Plus, she knew she'd have two cheerleaders in the office.

In 2015, Megan committed to running five days a week, every week, for a minimum of thirty minutes. At the time, given her foot issue, it seemed like an aggressive goal. But guess what? Once she found the right pair of shoes for her situation and resolved to run through the discomfort, the rest fell into place.

I don't have to tell you how this story ends but I will anyway. Fast forward seven years, and Megan's running streak lives on. She's had her fair share of challenges, including a pesky and frustrating sciatica issue, but she keeps going. She typically runs four times per week for three miles, plus one longer run of six to ten miles. This is someone who didn't think she could run at all and she's consistently outdoing me! She explains, "I'm not a runner. I just run." My thoughts exactly.

Megan and I aren't on the same team at work anymore, a sad and unfortunate fact of life, but her running streak remains alive and well. Why? Because although the daily encouragement and talk in the office was helpful, she made a commitment to herself that she refuses to break. That is the Power of the Streak.

My friend Phillip, who also happens to be my boss's son, has his own five-year workout streak. Phillip started his when he was in undergraduate school, and despite skepticism from his friends, he kept it alive through college and law school. He's now a busy prosecutor in a large city, and the streak lives on. That's no easy feat.

Are you sensing a pattern here? I really didn't until talking to friends and my husband while researching for this book. But interestingly, everyone in my inner circle who has committed to the streak and actually put in the effort to carry it out has kept it going indefinitely.

I realize that this sample size is extremely small, but it covers a wide range of ages and phases of life. It is a testament to the effectiveness of the streak concept to keep you working out no matter your age, walk of life, or personal circumstances. The streak doesn't discriminate. It can apply to a beginner, or to a professional athlete, and it can cut across all levels of athletic ability and experience. Powerful stuff.

3 TOO MUCH PRESSURE?

It doesn't even take a skeptic to ask whether committing to a workout streak puts too much pressure on yourself. What if life really is too busy? What if you legitimately try but you falter because of reasons outside your control? Will you become too obsessed with the idea of keeping the streak alive, to the exclusion of other things that are more important to you?

As for the first question, no one is too busy to commit to maintaining a baseline fitness level. Not even the President. If you think you are, ask yourself how long you plan to live the way you're currently living. Really—how long will you be able to maintain your current level of health without some form of regular exercise in your life? And by the time you realize you need to start regularly exercising, will your health have gotten to a point where starting will feel like an insurmountable challenge? We all know people who have gotten to this point. It's painful to watch, and more painful to live. You owe it to yourself to get ahead of it.

Next question: what about faltering because of reasons truly outside your control? Undoubtedly, this could happen. You could be involved in a serious car accident. You could be bitten by a random dog on a run. You could injure yourself—even with a simple look to the left (those of you in your late thirties and beyond know what I'm talking about). Any one of these events could end your streak.

The natural tendency is to believe that if the streak ends, you've necessarily failed. Game over. But if something outside your control does happen to cause your streak to end, you won't have failed. You'll have succeeded.

If my streak ends tomorrow, I will smile knowing that I made it more than twelve years of maintaining the running streak. I'm proud of it now, and I'll continue to be proud of it then. And you know what, as soon as I'm able, I'll start another streak. Why? Because by now, the streak is part of my makeup. It's part of my DNA. A temporary break in the streak won't alter that.

We'll talk more in Part Three about how to deal with injuries and setbacks. But the mere possibility of faltering should not deter you from starting a streak in the first place.

As for the third question: will the streak become too important or overtake your priorities? The answer to this question comes down to how you define your streak. We'll talk in detail about how to set the parameters in Part Two. For now, let's briefly study my streak requirements to figure out whether it's too much of a priority in my busy life.

My streak requires me to run a minimum of a mile for five days per week. A mile takes between eight and twelve minutes, depending on my fitness level, the weather, if I'm feeling particularly lazy, etc. So to keep my streak alive, I have to run a maximum of twelve minutes a day out of 1440 total minutes. And I get to choose two days per week that I don't have to do that at all.

Is my streak a priority? Absolutely. Is it too much of a priority? Absolutely not.

Some naysayers may question whether I really have a streak at all since I don't work out every single day of my life. I say, "*Seriously??*" I've run a minimum of five out of seven days for more than 600 weeks in row. That's streak worthy, even to a serial cynic. The beauty of the streak is that it is personal to you. It's all in how you define it.

I knew that if I committed to running every single day of my life, I'd be setting myself up for failure. That task seemed too daunting from the outset. I needed to know I'd have a break every once in a while. Others might feel the need to commit to every day so there are no breaks in the action or space for wiggle room. Still others might think five days a week is too much and opt for something less.

As long as you clearly define your streak in a way that will work for you long term, the streak will not overtake your life, I promise. Now, can I promise that you won't get the bug to do more? To run an organized run? Even a half or full marathon? No. But would that be so bad? I still have a hard time believing I've done the organized runs, but once I became fit in the running sense, I wanted to challenge myself in another way. Training for organized runs helped me meet that challenge. More about inspiration beyond the streak will follow in Part Four.

For now, keep in mind that even if getting that urge to do more than the minimum of the streak temporarily overtakes your priorities, it isn't the streak that is causing you to rebalance. Your streak is a *minimum*. A baseline. It may inspire you to do more than required, but it won't in itself cause you to reprioritize your life to the exclusion of other things that are important.

In the end, while it is perfectly normal to ask whether a workout streak is too much pressure for yourself, the reality is that if done correctly, a streak takes the pressure away. It provides a level of comfort because you know that you will have fitness and corresponding health without fail. It also gives you a daily or weekly "win," which can be hard to come by.

If I still haven't convinced you that a streak is not too much pressure on yourself, I have a middle ground that surely isn't. Try a streak for thirty days. We'll call it the "thirty-day streak challenge." Commit to the streak for one month of your life. See how it works. See how you feel. Decide if it feels like too much pressure. What do you have to lose? Think of it as a "try before you buy" situation.

At the end of the thirty-day streak challenge, decide if you want to keep the streak alive. Determine if you need to make some tweaks to keep it going long term. I'm confident that if you appropriately define your streak requirements and parameters, it will not feel like too much pressure, and you'll happily keep it going after thirty days. If, at the end of thirty days, it does feel like too much pressure, then you have been overly aggressive in defining your streak requirements. You'll need to adjust.

In the next part of this book, we will discuss the ins and outs of starting a streak and defining your streak requirements. I'll give you a number of exercise options and the pros and cons for each idea. We'll talk about the importance of setting a minimum amount of exercise to keep the streak alive—one that cannot be tinkered or fudged with in any way. We'll discuss the everyday approach versus the certain number of days each week approach. Last, we'll talk about the importance of having a target time of day for exercise along with why being flexible in carrying it out is also important.

PART TWO:

STARTING A STREAK

4 DEFINE YOUR EXERCISE REQUIREMENT

If I've convinced you to join me on this wild streak ride, or at least you're intrigued enough to think about it, the first step you'll need to take is deciding what type of exercise you will do for your streak. This could seem like a simple, no-need-to-think-about-it kind of task, especially if you recall that my decision was made because I was lazy and running seemed easy.

I recommend being more thoughtful than I was about what you'll do for your streak. Plus, I was probably a bit more thoughtful than I realized at the time. I knew I needed cardio to get in better shape. I saw the results my sister was getting by regularly running. I liked the idea of being outside rather than in a gym. I thought I could do it for free using nothing but the cheap old pair of tennis shoes in my closet (more on this later). There were probably other factors at play that I didn't even realize.

The single most important factor to think about when choosing what type of exercise is streak worthy for you is longevity. If you have back problems or knee problems or other residual injuries, you could be setting yourself up to fail if you choose an exercise that is high impact like running. If you've suffered a heart attack or other health problems, you could also be setting yourself up to fail if you are overly ambitious. Even if you have no residual injuries or health problems, you should not be too aggressive at the outset. Again, you have to think of something you can do every week without fail indefinitely. I hate to make this sound as important as naming your first-born child, but it's close.

This cannot be a phase. You can't decide you're sick of it after a couple of months and then want to do something else. No, you won't be married to the exercise in the sense that it's the only type you're able to do, but you will be doing at least this type of exercise indefinitely. Think of it as an open, rather than monogamous, marriage—you'll be forever loyal to the streak exercise but able to try others at the same time if your heart desires.

You also need to think about whether your chosen exercise requires equipment or something other than your body and some shoes to carry out. Why? Because if you commit to an exercise that requires heavy equipment (think elliptical) or a lap pool, you are likely to encounter some serious challenges when traveling or during holidays when gyms may be closed.

A natural question at this point is whether you have to commit to one particular type of exercise. What about just committing to doing "cardio" or "calisthenics"? (If you're unfamiliar with the concept of calisthenics, it's a form of working out that uses your body weight with little or no equipment and helps improve coordination, flexibility, and strength. Think pushups, jumping jacks, pull-ups, lunges, planks, etc.)

While I wouldn't foreclose entirely the idea of being more general with your exercise definition, I do think it's important to further define what will count. Two of the main ideas behind the streak are forced discipline and self-accountability. Being too general with the definition of your exercise could lead to a slippery slope because you could talk yourself into counting almost anything. For instance, will walking count as cardio? Will hiking? Dance? Chasing your toddler?

This is not to say that you won't be successful with the streak if you don't have a more specific exercise definition. My boss has had his exercise streak going for seventeen years and counting, and he defines the exercise requirement as "thirty minutes of aerobic exercise that is continuous and can be cycling, walking, running, or elliptical." My friend, Phillip, has a similar definition for his streak.

This more general method is doable, but not ideal. If you decide to take this route, I strongly suggest writing down a list of what "counts" in terms of exercise types within the general category you decide to pursue. You must stick to that list. Remember, you are doing this in part for self-accountability. You cannot give yourself any wiggle room in defining what counts. You can see that even though my boss's streak exercise requirement is "aerobic exercise," he has included a list of four exercises that actually count for this requirement.

To get the most overall fitness benefit from the streak exercise concept, I recommend you choose a cardio exercise (or exercises). Do not choose an exercise that requires someone else to accomplish. You must be dependent only on yourself and the necessary equipment to accomplish your exercise. Group sports are out. Tennis is out. The streak is an individual activity.

The list below contains six different cardio exercise options (running, elliptical, brisk walking, biking, swimming/water aerobics, and kickboxing), the equipment required, and some pros and cons of each from a streak perspective. This list is by no means comprehensive. You should be creative in thinking of something that will work for you, individually, for the long haul. If that means something not on the list or a combination of a few of these things, great!

There are so many resources for researching the various types of exercise and how to do them safely. I do not purport to be an expert in any of this, so I'll leave those topics to the experts. The list I've compiled is solely designed to help you brainstorm what you will choose.

And now for the overly obvious/lawyerly disclaimer: not everyone will be able to do all of the following exercises. If you have any doubt about your ability, please talk to your doctor before taking up something new. Remember, we are shooting for long-term health and fitness here, not an emergency room visit! Plus, please recall that I am an ordinary person with no expertise in fitness. If you need expert advice, consult an actual expert.

Finally, if you already know the type of exercise or exercises that you want to do and cannot be convinced otherwise, by all means, skip to the next chapter. Or, just read about the particular exercise(s) of interest to you. If you're on the fence, or open to other ideas, please read through each exercise listed. You might learn something new or get the urge to try one even if you don't think you will.

I'll start with running (or jogging) because I'm partial to it and know the most about it.

4.1 Running (or Jogging)

Running is great for strengthening your muscles, improving your cardiovascular fitness, burning those calories, and maintaining a healthy weight. Jogging is essentially a slower form of running with maybe slight alterations that really aren't relevant here. For the purposes of this discussion, I'll refer to it all as running.

One of the biggest pros to running is that you can run anytime, anywhere. You aren't dependent on anything except your shoes and GPS watch or timer. Heck, I've even done it in a pinch without any of that. You can choose the time of day, the place, and whether you have company. If you don't feel like bearing 95° heat in the summertime, you can do it inside, on a treadmill. You can even run in place if you're desperate.

As for the needed equipment, please, do me a favor and hear me out on running shoes. As usual, I was stubbornly slow to realize their importance, even when I was being begged to do so.

As I mentioned at the beginning of the book, when I started running, I literally grabbed an old pair of tennis shoes that had been gathering dust in my closet. Who knows how long I had them—since high school maybe? If I recall correctly, they were purchased because they were my favorite color (yellow) and looked cute. In other words, their ability to support an athletic activity was a non-factor.

A couple of weeks into my running journey, I noticed that my shins hurt quite a bit when I was running. I mentioned this to my boss, who immediately determined I had the wrong shoes, and told me exactly what I needed to do to get the right shoes. In typical "me" fashion, I balked at this advice. "Shoes cannot be that important. It must be something I'm doing or not doing. It'll pass."

I ran through the shin pain for a few months with my trusty and stylish, almost vintage, shoes. It got to a point that running even a mile became so painful that I considered quitting.

One day I rolled into the office, hustling to make it by 9:00 a.m., only to find a gift card placed on my chair. It was for the local running store. My boss, in his infinite wisdom, had figured out the true source of my resistance: I was being cheap. In other life areas, I was and remain overly extravagant with spending, but something about spending money on fitness didn't sit well. My boss knew if he gave me a gift card, I'd have no choice but to give new shoes a try.

The gift came with a few strings attached. I had to go to the running store, let them do the running test they do to figure out what "type" of runner I am, and pick a shoe based solely on comfort. I was not to worry about the brand or color or look. This was almost too much to ask of my mid-twenties self.

Since my boss was so generous and was truly trying to help, I drove to the running store with my marching orders, prepared to reluctantly carry them out. When I got there, I was met by a young employee who actually loved to run. His passion was palpable.

The running-store guy hooked me up to some machine and told me to run "normally" so he could see how my feet hit with each stride. I tried my best. After he diagnosed me, he asked, "What size are you?" "Eight and a half," I responded. "In running shoes?" Confused, I quipped, "Is there a special size system for running shoes I don't know about?" He just smiled and headed to the back.

When the young man returned, he had about six boxes of size TEN running shoes. Did he not hear me right? Did I not say it right? I asked him, "What's with the tens?" He then explained to his ignorant customer that it's crucial for a running shoe to let your toes breathe. You can't have your toes anywhere near touching the tops or fronts of the shoe. You should always get a size or so higher than your norm.

"But won't a size or size and a half up cause the shoe to float on my foot?" He again smiled and proceeded to tell me all the different ways you can tie your running shoe to avoid the floating problem.

I tried on every pair, jogged in place with each, and told him what I liked and didn't like in each one. Based on my comments, he brought out a few more pairs and we eventually narrowed it down to two options. The real me wanted the familiar brand that also looked cute. But alas, I chose for comfort as instructed.

I went home to try my first run in my new pair of shoes. To my complete surprise, my shin problem evaporated into thin air. It wasn't anything I was doing or not doing. It was my shoes.

Please, if you are going to run, go through the true running shoe buying experience. Visit your local running store. Not a place attached to a mall with a disinterested teenager talking to an invisible person (a/k/a concealed cellphone and AirPods) who is responsible for selling you the shoes. Go to a place where people live and breathe running. It will probably cost a little more, but it will be worth the extra money.

If they offer a diagnostic test, let them do it, no matter how strange it may feel. Size up. Try on different brands and styles. Wear different shoes on each foot and step in both. You are looking for the most comfortable shoe—the easiest way to find that is to compare them side-by-side. Your efforts will pay major dividends in pain-free running.

Once you know the best shoe for you, it becomes easier to buy them when you need to switch them out. Over the years, I've gone to a less cushioned model of the same brand of shoe but otherwise have kept consistent with the same brand and model every time. I know when I shop that I need to find this model and nothing else. If I'm lucky, I get to pick the color. But color is not a priority.

How long should running shoes be used? No, you should not run in the same pair until they fall apart. The general rule of thumb is that a running shoe should be replaced every 300 to 500 miles, when the midsole cushioning loses its resiliency. Personally, I now like to have three to four pairs at a time and rotate them out. That way, I'm regularly running with all different ages and wear levels of shoes. When it's time to retire one pair, I'm not shocked by having to break in a completely new pair for every run. I just add a new one into the rotation.

The only other crucial piece of equipment from a running perspective is a GPS watch or stopwatch. You guessed it: I initially used an old stopwatch. I was again being overly frugal and I didn't want to be discouraged by the true pace I was running. I much preferred "ball parking" it. A stopwatch is fine, but if your streak requires a certain distance, you may be giving yourself a little too much wiggle room by not tracking the actual mileage. For the first few years, I figured that I could run a mile in ten minutes, so if I was doing the minimum that day, I'd typically do about ten or eleven minutes.

A GPS, besides being a lot more affordable these days, offers a relatively reliable way to track your mileage. It can also offer other types of data such as your heart rate, the weather conditions, elevation levels, calories burned, and your pace per mile. This information can prove useful or overwhelming, depending on where you are on your streak journey. If you do use a GPS and you initially find yourself getting frustrated by the data, try opting for a simple stopwatch for a little while.

Although not necessary, a good pair of sunglasses will go a long way if you're running outside during daytime hours. I'm not talking about your favorite designer sunglasses. Trust me, I've tried running with those. The second you begin to sweat, those babies are sliding down your face. They become an extreme annoyance as you're pushing them back up every fourth stride.

There are all kinds of sunglasses out there that are made for sports specifically, but those types are not a must. You just need sunglasses that are lightweight and fit snugly on your face. My favorite pair of sunglasses for running were found sharing a junk drawer with mini screwdrivers, old toothpaste, and a retainer from circa 1994.

Other gear can include a hat and sunscreen if it's daytime. If you run at nighttime, or so early in the morning that it's still dark (props to you), please consider brightly-colored clothes or reflective tape. It could feel goofy, but runners can be difficult to see for people driving. Even if you're just running in your neighborhood, it's better to be safe than sorry.

A huge positive to running that I never expected is seeing new places in a different way. There's something exhilarating about exploring a new place on foot, outside a vehicle. Obviously, you have to do this with confidence that you're in an area that is safe. If you do though, it can really be great.

If it weren't for my streak, I can almost guarantee that I never *ever* would go for the idea of running while on vacation. I still have trouble with the idea. But sometimes the streak requires you to exercise while traveling, so I suck it up when necessary.

I've seen so much more of new cities and places while running that I'd likely never see otherwise. Sure, you can sight see quite a bit by walking, but running is different because you cover more than twice the ground in the same time period, and you are likely doing it without the whole family or group of friends traveling with you.

Have you ever run through Central Park in New York City? What about the National Mall in Washington, D.C.? Grant Park in Chicago? The grounds of the Biltmore estate in Asheville? Even the serial cynic is here to tell you there's something majestic about all these places in the quiet of the morning, pre-coffee and pre-toddler screams, hearing only the sounds of your feet hitting the ground and maybe a bird chirping here and there.

Running is also responsible for discovering unique places I otherwise wouldn't have found on trips. It could be a divine local bistro, a donut place that does you right, a new coffee shop, or something else. Running past these types of establishments gives you an opportunity to be more observant than you would be in a vehicle. If you see a donut joint with a line out the door and your mouth starts watering from the aromas as you pass, you know it's a must-do on the trip. Plus you can do it guilt-free knowing that you earned it.

Another positive of running is the mental health benefit. Have you heard of the "runner's high?" Described by healthline.com in an October 2020 article on the subject as a "brief, deeply relaxing state of euphoria," or "extreme joy or delight," this is the kind of thing that is typically experienced by the use of a controlled substance. You can get it naturally just by running!

Not everyone experiences the "runner's high." In fact, healthline.com speculates that it can be pretty rare. Because it's subjective and different for everyone, it's hard to tell how many actually get it. Unfortunately for me, I haven't. In fact, running most often feels like a serious chore for me—as bad as folding toddler laundry—even during my best runs. There is nothing euphoric about it.

I have, however, experienced significant mental health benefits from running, a relatable experience for most people. Running allows me to clear my mind and reset. Since I typically run in the evenings after work, it helps me decompress from a busy day. It's almost like a quick form of daily therapy.

There's a noticeable pattern of how my mind works during a run. The first several minutes, I think about nothing. I just let my mind clear of all the madness from the day. Maybe I'll observe a pretty yard or two.

If I'm only running the minimum of a mile, that's about where it ends. Afterwards, I feel more relaxed and excited to see my toddler banging at the front door and my six-year-old ready to tell me all about her daily star color.

If I'm running for three or more miles, my mind quiets for the first half, and then I start thinking about new ideas for the second, even if I'm not consciously trying. If I'm grappling with how to resolve a tough legal question at work, a creative resolution may come to me. If I'm worried about my children or my siblings, I'll brainstorm healthy ways to address my fears. If nothing in particular is bothering me, I could get a random idea that helps me in a seriously positive way. As I said before, running is even responsible for the idea of writing this book!

If I'm venturing past four or five miles, my mind switches from creative, problem-solving mode to survival mode. I start telling myself ways that I'll get through it. Pep talks, distance calculations, countdowns, you name it. Whatever gets me through. I don't know about you, but I am not one to give myself a pep talk in other areas of life. I'm actually way too self-critical and have a tendency to be negative about myself. Running a longer distance forces me to be nice to myself to get through it, a strong benefit from a mental health perspective. It gives me a break from me.

There are several cons to running, especially as a streak exercise. The biggest con from a longevity standpoint is that running can be hard on your body. Running is high impact and bears your whole weight. The stress from this impact can take quite a toll and can lead to injury. Important for avoiding injury are stretching before and after a run, allowing for adequate rest, and not over doing it. As with most cardio exercises, it's also important to stay hydrated.

Even with its high impact, running is a streak-worthy exercise. At the time of this writing, Jon Sutherland holds the record for a consecutive day one-mile running streak: more than 53 years. Lois Bastien holds the record for a female: more than 42 years. There are scores of people all over the planet who have consecutive day running streaks, ranging from one year to 53. With the right formula, an indefinite running streak is achievable.

Another con to running, at least outside, is the random jerk who thinks it's funny to honk at you, yell at you, or otherwise try to throw you off your game. Imagine being on mile five, thinking you could be on the brink of death, trying with all your might to convince yourself to make it just one more mile, when a car flies by and—HONK!!

Besides scaring the hell out of me every time, it's infuriating. My heart races, sometimes feeling like it will jump out of my chest. I involuntarily jump. Inevitably, the jerk rolls down the window and laughs as loud as he can to make sure I hear how pleased he is with himself (sorry, guys, but 95% of the time the culprit is a male).

I have never understood this behavior. Who actually thinks it's funny to do this? And why? Clearly, I have a bit of a complex on the subject. But I think it's with good reason. One guy actually had a horn that sounded like an airhorn—that was *the worst*.

Unfortunately, this honking craze is a strange fact of running. If I'm on a remotely busy road, I can count on at least two scare-the-hell-out-of-me moments a week. I've never learned how to get over it.

Random dogs and animals can also cause a scare. In my twelve years of running outside, through all different types of neighborhoods, I've had only three legitimate dog-chasing scares, and no actual attacks. I am not an animal hater, but I have developed an unhealthy animosity for people who let their large, aggressive dogs roam freely.

To combat the potentially-dangerous dog situation, I've recently decided to run with a small can of pepper spray. And of course it could also help defend against an unlikely human attack. I recommend you do the same.

Leave it to me to leave my favorite exercise topic on such a dim note! Even with its cons though, running remains my number one choice because of all the pros that I've outlined. And some of the challenges in running are going to be present with the other exercises listed below. Like with most irritants, there are ways to work around them and not let them overtake the benefits. If I had to choose my streak exercise all over again, I'd stick with running. If you are able, I hope you give it strong consideration.

4.2 Elliptical Machine

The elliptical is a stationary exercise machine that provides a low-impact cardio workout. The leg movements on an elliptical are designed to mimic running, walking, or cross-country skiing (to the extent possible) without the impact. Some ellipticals also have arm handles that move back and forth together with the foot platforms, which is great for providing a full-body workout. Elliptical machines come in all shapes and sizes, with varying prices and degrees of durability. You can buy your own, or you can find one at almost any gym these days.

An elliptical is a great alternative to running. Put simply, the elliptical workout is solid cardio but is easy on the joints. A win-win. Unlike running, you can go forwards or backwards on an elliptical. Surprisingly, I actually prefer backwards.

To work out on an elliptical machine, you'll need at least the machine itself and a great pair of shoes. See the previous section (4.1, Running) on the importance of shoes and how to go about picking them out.

On the pro side for the elliptical as a streak exercise, its low-impact, high-cardio workout is likely to give you solid results with corresponding longevity. Because the impact is not as hard as running, stress injuries are less likely. Also, you can typically choose from a variety of exercise options on the machine, including hill climbing and interval training.

An elliptical is almost always stationed inside, so you'll have a perfectly cool (or warm) environment for your workout. Another big pro to using the elliptical is that you can actually read or use an iPad or watch television or whatever else while doing it (reading is a little tricky, but doable). Multitasking is always a plus!

The largest con for doing the elliptical as your streak exercise is obvious: you need access to the machine to do it. If you have one at home or decide to purchase one, that will easily take care of the availability factor while you are home. Be sure to put it in an area of your house where you won't be disturbing anyone by using it. Our elliptical is currently in our bedroom. Not the best choice. If my husband goes to bed at 9:00 p.m. and I want to do a late-night workout, I'm out of luck.

Avoid putting up unnecessary barriers to your being able to do your streak exercise whenever you want or need to do it.

If you don't buy a machine, you'll need to use one at the gym. Warning: the elliptical is *very* popular at the gym. It is not uncommon to have to wait to use one, which can be discouraging, especially because you won't be able to substitute something else that happens to be available to count for your streak. If you don't currently have a gym and are shopping around for one to join, you'll want to check how many elliptical machines the gym has and ask about their popularity.

Having an elliptical at home or at the gym likely covers the vast majority of your time, but what about traveling? These days, most hotels have some sort of gym, and if the gym is larger than a closet and has more than two obligatory machines, chances are it'll have an elliptical. But that is not guaranteed. You can always call a hotel in advance to check. Also, if you are a member of a gym that has multiple locations or the YMCA, you can often attend the gym or Y in your traveling destination as a guest.

Besides a hotel, you could find yourself on a cruise ship. Little known fact among cruisers: cruise ships have gyms! Every cruise ship I've been on has a relatively large gym that includes multiple elliptical machines.

What about camping though? Or staying out of town with friends who don't own an elliptical and don't live near a gym? Depending on the length of these trips and your weekly streak requirements, these kinds of experiences could cause your streak to be in serious jeopardy if you choose the elliptical, and only the elliptical, as your streak exercise.

Some criticize the elliptical by claiming it is too easy. I think it's true that the elliptical *can be* too easy, which can create serious challenges to getting and staying fit. For instance, I can say I'm getting on the elliptical for thirty minutes and actually do that, but if my speed is less than I would do walking, how much of a workout am I actually getting?

It's all up to you to decide whether you are working out hard enough on an elliptical. If you aren't, it's up to you to push yourself to work harder. The machine will give you estimates on how many calories you've burned and how many miles you've gone, so you'll have some objective measure of how you're doing. But, if you know you are the type of person to take the easy way out, the elliptical may not be for you.

Even with its faults, the elliptical is a solid choice, especially if you want great cardio but have an existing injury or health issue that makes running not possible or attractive.

4.3 Brisk Walking

Walking is seriously underrated as exercise. Achievable by most people, brisk, regular walking can help you maintain healthy weight, lose body fat, prevent or manage health conditions, improve cardiovascular fitness, increase your energy levels, help your mood and sleep, improve balance, and even reduce stress, according to MayoClinic.org. The more briskly and more regularly you walk, the more you benefit.

Equipment needed is similar to running: a great, comfortable pair of shoes (see the Running section, 4.1, on picking these out) and a timer or GPS. If you're walking during the day, you'll want sunscreen, sunglasses, and maybe a hat. At night, opt for bright colors or reflective tape.

What you need to remember if you choose walking as your exercise is that you are doing it for the exercise. A brisk pace, or working up to one, is important. I'm not talking about a walking-your-new-puppy type of pace. No stopping to chase lizards or smell the roses. No stopping to check your text messages or getting your two-year-old out of the stroller for a toddler-paced walk. At least for your designated time or distance to maintain your streak, you've got to move with a brisk pace that *feels* like the workout it was meant to be. After that time, sure, get the toddler out. One of the great benefits to walking as a streak exercise is the ability to do it with a stroller or older children or your spouse or anyone!

Another big benefit to walking is that you can do it anytime, anywhere, and wearing anything. Yes, comfy workout clothes and shoes are must-haves for the day-to-day routine but in a pinch, you could walk without those things if you find yourself forgetting them.

Too hot outside? Storming outside? Forgot to walk until 10:00 p.m. when kids are asleep and husband or wife is gone? No problem. Walk on a treadmill if you have one. Walk inside your house repeating the same pattern 100 times if need be. Have you ever tried to walk round and round inside the house with small kids who are awake? Inevitably, they end up chasing after you and giggling. You can turn a less-than-ideal situation into a fun game! Or maybe you'll purposely opt for the 10:00 p.m. indoor walk to save your sanity for the evening.

The obvious point here is that walking is achievable in almost any condition. Also, walking carries less risk of injury, making it ideal from a streak longevity standpoint. Just make sure when you're walking outside that you're staying vigilant about changes in sidewalk heights. You don't want to trip on a raised sidewalk and take yourself out. (Yes, I'm speaking from experience here.)

A con to walking as your streak exercise is that you won't get as much of a cardio workout as you would with most exercise forms. But again, a brisk walk will go a long way on this front. Also, walking is a great way to get started if you don't currently exercise. Remember, you can always build your way up to something more. The focus for now should be choosing something that is achievable long term.

Another con to walking, depending on where you're doing it, is the possibility of jerks honking their horns to scare you (I talked about these people in the Running section).

Probably the biggest con to walking as a streak exercise is that it simply takes longer to get a decent workout. You can cover twice the ground or more in the same amount of time by running if you're able. Certainly more time is not a deal breaker, but if you are pressed for time already, it's something to consider. For instance, if your streak requires you to walk one mile per day, you are likely going to spend approximately eighteen to twenty minutes doing it. Really not much in the scheme of things, but to get a solid workout from walking, you may need to increase your mileage to more than one a day. This will result in more time spent.

All in all, walking is highly versatile and highly effective when done regularly and well. It's a great option.

4.4 Biking (or Cycling)

Regular biking is great for improving your body strength and providing a low-impact cardio workout. It also helps you with balance. You can ride a stationary bike at home or in the gym, alone or via a class (a virtual class if at home), or you can opt for the old-fashioned method of cycling outdoors on a bike, alone or with a group (a real peloton!).

The most important piece of equipment for biking is the bike itself. If you opt for a stationary bike at home, there is no shortage of available options on the market. Some stationary bikes come with subscriptions, where you pay a monthly fee to have access to all sorts of different virtual classes, both live and recorded. You can also opt for solitary rides through multitudes of virtual reality lands. Some stationary bike subscription services even keep track of your streak!

Stationary bikes come in all sizes and at all price points. You'll want to research the different options, check reviews, and find one that will work best for you for the long haul.

If you are choosing to do the stationary bike at a gym, you'll want to check what types of bikes are available and see how popular they are. If you choose to bike on the road, you'll need a bike that is made for exercising. You don't want to use your cute beach bike. A good road bike, made mostly for riding on pavement, has an aerodynamic design that will be more comfortable for longer periods. These bikes are designed to go far and fast. That is what you want in a workout bike. Other options include mountain bikes— best for trails and rocky roads—or hybrid bikes that are suitable for all different types of terrain.

Like stationary bikes, those designed for riding outside come at various price points and are carried by all sorts of retailers. Going to a local cycling shop will prove to be a great education for the different types and styles available.

Another solid option is purchasing a bike for cycling outside, and also purchasing a piece of equipment for turning it into a stationary bike at home. There are various models of this type of equipment on the market. This method allows you to ride the same bike all the time, but you have the choice of riding it inside or outside.

Other equipment needed for cycling includes tight "bike" shorts—if you can stand them—to cut down on resistance and make for a more comfortable riding experience (otherwise, opt for anything that isn't too loose), a helmet, sunglasses for keeping the sun out of your face and bugs out of your eyes, and appropriate shoes. If you have a true road bike, you may need a special type of shoe that "clicks in" to the pedals. This makes pedaling a better experience because you don't have to worry about your foot sliding off. Your local cycling shop can help you through the ins and outs of cycling shoes. Also, you may opt for a pair of cycling gloves to keep a better grip on the handlebars.

On the pro side of cycling from a streak viewpoint, it's a great workout and is low impact, carrying less risk of injury from a stress perspective. If you suffer knee or back problems, however, long-term cycling may not be for you. The position you ride a bike in can be very strenuous on your back. Also, the constant pedaling motion can be a challenge for knee issues.

Continuing on the pro side, cycling can be done *almost* anywhere. If you're more of a stationary bike person, I like the option of purchasing a less expensive hybrid bike for the road, just in case. Think about camping trips or day trips.

If you're a road-bike person, you may have to be prepared to use a stationary bike when traveling, in places like hotels. However, with the advent of the city-bike sharing programs, you may not even need to do that. Plus, what a great way to explore a new city: by bike! As we discussed in the Running section (4.1), working out while exploring is really a win-win.

Another great pro to biking is that it can get you from point "A" to point "B." This means you can use your streak exercise to accomplish multiple things. You can bike to work and back. You can bike to your friend's house for dinner. You can bike to the park with kids in tow (they'll love it!). It's a fun and simple way to transport yourself.

On the con side of biking as a streak exercise is that while you can do it almost anywhere, you do have to have access to one. Another con to road biking is the potential danger. If you don't have a good biking trail nearby, chances are you'll find yourself on the actual road quite a bit. With the proliferation of distracted driving as of late, being on the road often means a higher chance of being hit by a car. Riding in a group (peloton style) greatly reduces this risk. Also, wearing reflective tape helps. Use a biking lane whenever possible. Make sure you're paying close attention to traffic and others around you.

Road biking also carries a risk of falling off the bike and injuring yourself. Staying vigilant about your surroundings reduces the risk of falling because you are less likely to be surprised and have to react quickly.

Outdoor cycling is not an exercise that is good for multitasking!

In the end, cycling is a great activity and a solid choice as a streak exercise.

4.5 Swimming or Water Aerobics

Swimming and water aerobics are great forms of exercise. Both help with cardiovascular health, joint health, muscular endurance, and strength building. Plus, being in a pool literally means being cool!

Swimming in particular is very low impact and is a great full-body workout. Common strokes include the breaststroke, backstroke, side stroke, freestyle, and butterfly. Each has its own unique set of challenges and benefits. Swimming is best performed in a pool designed for it: a lap pool. This is a longer-length pool that is designed to optimize your workout from each lap before you turn around and go on to the next one.

Water aerobics are usually performed with the person standing about waist deep in a pool. It can be any pool, but one with about waist deep water for at least a portion works best. Exercises often include running in the pool, jumping, strength training, arm work, ab work, and kicking. The water naturally resists every move you make, causing your body to gain flexibility and mobility. Water resistance also serves to better tone your muscles but is not so great for building lean muscle mass. Since you are in water, you don't have to worry about falling if you lose your balance. Plus, since you're under water, people can't really tell if you misstep—this makes for a less judgy group workout experience.

For water aerobics, you'll want a good pair of water shoes so you can have some traction on the bottom of the pool. Many water aerobics classes use foam dumbbells, possibly a buoyancy belt, and maybe some resistance gloves. These gloves are webbed and make for even more resistance in the water. You'll want to pick up at least some foam dumbbells if you're exercising at home, or ask your gym if the necessary equipment is provided.

If your eyes are sensitive to chlorine, you'll want a good pair of goggles for swimming or water aerobics. Although you typically don't submerge your whole body for water aerobics, it is not uncommon to splash the water, so you could find it landing in your eyes. Some also choose to wear a swim cap for swimming and water aerobics. This helps keep your hair chlorine-free. If you are in the pool often for your streak exercise, your hair will thank you for some cap protection. Or, if you're like my husband and don't mind the natural bleach effect, leave the cap off. Remember when "dying the tips" was cool? Yep, we are bringing it back.

Seriously though, if chlorine sensitivity is a problem for you, these are not your ideal streak exercises. Unfortunately for me, I've developed a big sensitivity to the smell of chlorine as I've otherwise gracefully aged. This sensitivity, combined with a seriously aggressive chlorine policy at my husband's gym, dictates an immediate shower for him every time he walks in the door from working out. Let's be honest, he could use one anyway.

On the pro side for swimming and water aerobics as streak exercises are their low impact, high cardio, full-body workouts. As Tyler's story shows, swimming is an ideal exercise for someone who suffers from back problems. A good swimming workout can also be accomplished in a relatively short period of time—similar to a benefit of running. As well, it's hard to "cheat" while swimming because you have to go a certain speed and make enough movement to stay afloat, and you know exactly how many laps you need to accomplish to keep the streak alive.

A big con of both swimming and water aerobics for anyone with body image issues is getting in a bathing suit. Obviously if you have your own pool and can do it alone, this won't be as much of an issue. But going to the gym in a bathing suit can make even a relatively fit person squirm. I'm here to tell you, though, that most people doing water aerobics classes at gyms are very welcoming and not judgy. Plus, you can robe up until the last minute and quickly slip into the pool if needed. Try not to let the bathing suit factor deter you if you're otherwise interested in these options.

Another con of these exercises is the requirement of having an accessible pool. If you have a pool at home that fits the requirements for swimming or water aerobics, this is not as big of an issue for you, but you still have to figure out what you'll do when traveling. Even if you have access to a hotel pool, do you want to be the random person in the corner doing water aerobics? Personally, I'm at a point of not exactly minding how this would look to strangers I'll never see again—maybe it would detract from the six-year-old's cannonballs—but you may not be there.

Aside from the perception issues being a possible challenge on vacations, my husband and I have learned that there are certain times when a pool that is large enough for swimming laps just won't be available to you. For example, the pool on a cruise ship is too tiny and too full of partiers to be a candidate for swimming laps. If you were desperate though, maybe you could go early in the morning right when it opens and just deal with the constant back and forth in the name of the streak. Another option is swimming at a port, which typically has some body of water—ocean, pool, etc. You may have to get creative.

If you choose to swim or do water aerobics at a gym for your everyday workout, you'll want to see how many swim lanes are available and how popular they are. It is not uncommon to have to wait for a swimming lane at a gym. For water aerobics, you'll want to check available class times and also check whether you're permitted to do them on your own in the pool(s) for times when you aren't able to make a class. You have to have a backup plan for unexpected cancellations or alterations in class times or your schedule. You cannot be dependent solely on the class.

All in all, swimming and water aerobics can be great exercise and streak achievable with the right commitment.

4.6 Kickboxing

Kickboxing is a form of martial art. It is a total-body workout that includes punching, jabbing, and kicking. Kickboxing is very high impact and keeps your heart rate high as well. It's great for improving your balance, flexibility, and strength. Kickboxing is usually taught in a class at a martial arts studio or gym, but you can do the moves on your own as well through apps, streaming, or retro DVDs.

Necessary gear for kickboxing includes gloves and the equipment you will punch and kick. Generally, kickboxing is done barefoot or with socks, but some gyms allow you to wear shoes such as cross trainers.

Equipment can also include hand and ankle wraps, a mouthguard, headgear, and shin guards.

A big pro of kickboxing that isn't as present in the other exercises we've discussed is that it can greatly help with confidence and self-esteem. Plus, it helps with self-defense.

Another big pro is that it could be the single best exercise we've discussed for mental health, probably even better than running. Imagine the feelings of relief you'd have by regularly punching and kicking in an environment where these things are encouraged! After a long day of work or dealing with kids, you can go to kickboxing class or put in a DVD at home and *have at it*.

A con to kickboxing is the high-impact total-body workout leads to more possibility of injury, particularly muscle strains. However, the workout targets overall body strength, so if you are not overdoing it, your body should become stronger over time and able to handle the stress of the workout. The key here is to ease into it if you're a beginner.

If you choose to take a kickboxing class, a big con from a streak perspective will be that you'll have to work out at a set time of day. Also, if you go out of town, you'll have a hard time getting your workout in. I'd suggest having the necessary equipment and a DVD or app readily available at home for those times when you just can't make it to class, the gym is closed, or for when you need to go out of town. Obviously you can't travel with a punching or boxing bag if you're flying, so you'll need to get creative on how you deal with that obstacle.

All in all, kickboxing is a fun and great idea for a streak exercise.

4.7 Final Thoughts on the Exercise to Choose

I hope the above list has given you some good ideas for the type of exercise that will be best for you in the long term. If nothing has resonated, then be more creative than I have been! The list is not meant to be exhaustive or exclusive. In the end, you need to choose something that is right for you and your lifestyle. If that means a combination of exercises or something not even on the list, by all means go for it. Just commit to whatever it is and stick with it.

5 SET YOUR MINIMUM MILEAGE, LAPS, OR TIME

By now, you should have chosen the exercise or exercises you'll do for your streak. Equally important is choosing the minimum amount of mileage, laps, or time you will do to make the activity "count" for the day.

In setting your minimum, you must avoid being too aggressive. I'm reminded of a recent, leisurely bike ride I took with my sister and a great family friend while visiting Cape Cod. About fifteen minutes into the ride, my sister asked me, "Are you glistening yet?" I responded, "Yep, I'm glistening." She quipped back, "Okay, we've done enough." This story, besides perfectly summing up the max effort any normal person would want to put into exercising during a nice vacation, should be your starting point for thinking about your minimum. Why? Because the goal here is not to commit to doing a full workout every single time. The goal is to glisten, to commit to doing your streak exercise with enough mileage, laps, or time to have felt like you did *something*, but not *everything*.

Remember, you have to do your streak exercise when you're feeling tired, worn down, and even sick. I chose a mile because I know I can almost surely run a mile no matter how I'm feeling. Had I chosen two or three miles as my minimum, that would feel much more difficult and maybe even impossible to accomplish if I'm feeling ill or even just over it. When I'm feeling bad and need to run to keep the streak alive, I say to myself, "I can do anything for ten minutes." It's true, you can.

A good question here is whether doing something for as little as ten minutes or a mile is worth it. Yes, it most certainly is, because the minimum you choose to keep your streak alive is not what you'll do every single time. Sure, doing only your streak minimum day in and day out may not cause an Insta-worthy transformation, but it keeps the exercise going. It gives you a baseline of fitness and confidence that is worth the effort.

Some days, you'll have the urge and motivation to do more; other days you won't. For instance, I ran eight miles today because the weather conditions were right, I wanted to get at least one longer run in this week, and I could force myself to do it by running home from my sister's house. But tomorrow and the next day will probably be minimum one-mile days, or even days off, to allow for recovery and rest.

If you don't set the bar too high with your minimum, you should be able to do your exercise even through minor illness or injury. This is important because it ensures you won't have a few bad days and decide to do nothing, only to lose motivation to exercise at all. Instead, you will have a few minimum days that don't feel great but you persist anyway and you know your streak is alive. When you do feel better or more motivated, you will do more.

The difference here is powerful. A few days completely off can translate into serious motivation kill even when you are feeling better. A few days of feeling bad but keeping the streak alive means when you are feeling better, you will have motivation to do more. It's literally the difference between doing *nothing* and doing *more than something*.

This is not to say you won't be successful if you choose to do more than I have. My boss, my friend Phillip, and my friend Megan all chose to do a minimum of thirty minutes for their streak exercises. But Phillip, who had a setback of a bad illness that ended his original streak, explains that the illness helped him realize he couldn't go "90 to nothing" every day. Rather, there has to be a good balance so that the streak can adapt to life as much as possible. You have to choose something that is right for you and something you are confident you can do even when you're not feeling motivated or particularly well.

Avoiding an overly aggressive minimum amount also helps you get through the days when you have every intention of having a great workout, but after you get going you just aren't feeling it. I can't tell you how many times I've laced up thinking I'm going to set the world on fire with my mileage, only to feel terrible from the outset and stop after one. It has to be in the hundreds. My two pregnancies come to mind for some serious consecutive one-mile days. Just as well, there are times when I lace up thinking I'll be doing the one-mile minimum, only to get outside and feel good enough to keep going beyond that one mile.

In setting your minimum, I recommend using mileage, laps, or the like whenever possible. I like using these markers, rather than time because these markers force a certain amount of physical exercise. For instance, if I set ten minutes—rather than a mile—as my minimum, I could run at an absolute snail's pace for ten minutes and call it a day. Forcing myself to do a mile means that I'm going to run that mile whether it takes me eight minutes or fifteen. It incentivizes me to get it done quicker, especially if I'm doing the minimum that day. This means a better workout, even if it is just a minimum day. The same could be said for doing miles—rather than a certain amount of time—on a bike, walking, on the elliptical, and doing laps in a pool.

If you are choosing to do multiple exercises that count, it may or may not be possible to set a minimum that is not time dependent. Kickboxing and water aerobics are exercises that may be tough for carrying out this idea.

If you do choose time as your measure, you should consider having a requirement to get your heart rate up to a certain level—whatever you decide—for it to count as your minimum for the day. You can measure your heart rate via a monitor, some GPS watches, Apple watches, and the like. Determine your desired heart rate and ensure that you are getting that level during your allotted time.

Another consideration for your minimum amount of exercise per day is whether the mileage or time needs to be consecutive, or whether it can be broken up. I recommend making the requirement consecutive. For me, one consecutive mile means I set out to run, I know I have to do it for a mile, and then it is done for the day. If you allow yourself to do less than the minimum per session, it could actually be a disservice to you because it will feel like more work to have to start exercising two or more times in one day. Just set the minimum, make it consecutive, and go for it. If you have a particularly chatty mail-person or neighbor who stops you mid-run once in a blue moon, that is okay. Reset your GPS and start again right then and there or start over later in the day if you must.

If you are just beginning with regular exercise, you should be very conservative in setting your minimums. A good rule of thumb for running is one mile, for walking is one to two miles, for the elliptical is one mile, for biking is five miles, and for swimming is ten laps.

If you are choosing to take a class or classes as part of your streak exercise, obviously you'll need to do the length of the class most of the time, but you could think about setting your minimum at just ten to fifteen minutes for those times when you have to squeeze in the workout without getting to or taking a whole class. Kickboxing and water aerobics, which are generally more dependent on classes, require more time per session than the other recommended exercises, so you may want to think about making your weekly requirement less for these exercises (probably three days per week).

If you already exercise some and are confident in your ability to do more than what I've suggested, by all means go for it. Just remember to think long term. Not how you feel right now or how you'll feel a few months from now. This is a long-term marriage—not a fun fling.

Keep in mind that something that works for this particular phase of your life may not always work for other phases. If you are conservative with your minimum now, you will have less chance of having to redefine your streak requirements later. If you're in your twenties and have all the energy and strength in the world (except after Thirsty Thursdays), that same energy may not follow you into your thirties after several all-nighters with a restless baby, or after staying at the office until midnight trying to meet a deadline. The same could be said for any stage of life.

You should aim to choose a minimum amount that is adaptable to all eras and life circumstances. At the end of the day, this decision is very personal to you just like every other aspect of your streak.

6 SET YOUR MINIMUM DAYS PER WEEK

The next step is to set the minimum number of days per week that you will exercise. Are you the type of person who wants or needs to work out every day to keep a streak alive, or will you want or need some days off? There is no right or wrong answer.

As I mentioned before, I chose five days per week because I needed to know I would have a couple days off. But it still felt very substantial in terms of days spent with some amount of working out. Partly because I was doing so many days per week, I kept my mileage requirement low. Another, almost opposite, approach would be to make a higher minimum exercise requirement but a lower days-per-week requirement.

You need to take into account your *realistic* lifestyle, not your *ideal* lifestyle, in deciding the number of days per week you know you can work out. If you lead a very busy life and have a spouse and children, figure out how many days per week you can get away and/or bring the kids with you to work out.

Obviously, you'll need support from your spouse some days. My husband and I know that we have to work around each other's schedules to a degree to get our exercising in for the day. On weekends, if we need to run or swim to keep our respective streaks alive, we help each other out by taking turns watching the kids. But when he is not around, I figure it out by either taking the kids with me or sending them to a family member for a little bit. My six-year-old can now run a mile consistently, and my one-year-old enjoys cheering us on from the stroller. If you are committed, you can find a way. You just have to be practical about it.

In setting your minimum number of days per week, I recommend at least three. Doing something only two out of seven days per week doesn't feel like a regular, consistent activity. It's easy to lose track of the last day you exercised if multiple days can pass in between. Plus, the gurus will tell you that the benefits of exercising two days per week are not nearly as good as opting for at least three or four days.

The type of exercise you'll be doing should also inform the decision on the number of days per week you'll commit to it. Those exercises we've discussed with minimal roadblocks or equipment needed—mainly running and walking—are easier to do more often or even every day. The elliptical, biking, swimming, water aerobics, and kickboxing could be more challenging to do every single day.

Also think about how often you travel and whether you want working out to be an essential part of your travel. If you often take long weekends away or are going away on business for two or three days, you can opt to make your streak week four out of seven days so that you are not forced to exercise while traveling.

Sure, it will require you to work out more often while at home, but you'll have the option to choose not to on the road. Options are good.

I applaud those who work out every single day of their lives. That takes serious commitment. While it may seem like a lot of pressure to commit to every single day, those who do it seem to take comfort in exercise being an essential part of each and every day. Sleep, eat, drink, and work out. It could be that simple. My friend, Phillip, tells me that it grounds him knowing that he finished his daily workout.

Plus, if you opt for running and choose to do it every day, there are actual registries for people who have daily running streaks. A public declaration of your streak's beginning and progress made would be an additional incentive to keep the streak alive!

Another question you need to answer—if you don't choose the every-day approach—is what day of the week does your streak week start? This may sound silly, but it's actually pretty important for ensuring you are getting your minimum number of days under your belt. I started my streak on Memorial Day, which falls on a Monday. So, I have Monday through Sunday to run five days.

Although it was sheer chance that dictated the Monday start day for me, I like it this way—I know going into the weekend whether I need to run two of the days, one of the days, or none at all based on my weekday performance. If I had chosen to start my week on Saturday, however, I would likely blow off exercising all weekend and go into the following week knowing I've got a lot of work to do. That would feel awfully heavy. This example shows that picking a certain day to start your week can make significant differences in mindset, intended or not. It's deserving of attention like picking the day and time of your college classes (8:00 a.m. on Friday: hard pass) or maintaining your child's social calendar. A little strategy is in order.

That about sums up the important considerations for setting your days-per-week requirement. If it feels like you've had to make a lot of important decisions at this point, I get it. But you've got to be thoughtful at this beginning stage to ensure longevity. Once you make these decisions, the rest falls into place and your brain essentially goes on autopilot when it comes to working out.

7 SET YOUR TARGET WORKOUT TIME OF DAY

You've now made all the important, must make, streak decisions. Congrats! The next step in starting your streak is to set a target time of day for your workout. Unlike the other decisions you've made so far which shouldn't have any room for flexibility once your streak starts, this one *requires* you to be flexible. It's a target for a reason. Life won't always allow you to work out at the same time each day. So you have a plan, but you can change it as circumstances dictate. The best thing about a plan is being able to change it.

Anyone who knows me knows that I have a problem with rage in the mornings. I've always been this way, and probably always will. I just don't do mornings. This was a very manageable flaw in early adulthood, but with kids it's tricky. Add on a husband who leaves before the rest of us wake up each morning, it's even trickier. Each day that I get myself out of bed, take a shower, make two lunches, get the kids out of bed, clothe them, feed them, brush all teeth, and deliver them to required places on time with minimal incidents is a serious win.

I tell you this about myself to make the point that if I chose to work out in the morning, I'd last approximately one day. Seriously. I knew that going in. So when I decided (waaaaaay pre-children) to start the streak, I knew my target time of day would have to be after work.

Exercising after work has its own challenges because it goes without saying that after a long day, I just want to unwind, rest, and stream something meaningless on TV. For that reason, I initially decided I would run from the office before leaving for home each day. Besides having a built-in running partner (my boss), doing it this way ensured that I would, in fact, do it. Another added benefit was letting rush hour traffic dissipate while I was running. Because of the traffic benefit, even if I took an extra half hour at the end of the day to run, the reality was that I would only get home ten to fifteen minutes later because I wouldn't be stuck in traffic. Not a bad trade off.

As time has passed, I still run after work, but not always from the office anymore. I've now gained enough self-trust to be able to drive home and run from there, or drive to my favorite running trail on the way home. But the key is that I always bring my running clothes to work and change before I leave. This simple routine is important because if I've already taken the time to change into workout clothes, I'm not going to waste an opportunity to run once I leave the office. By contrast, if I didn't bring clothes to the office, I'd have to make it home every day, change, and then go out. I'd have a bunch more roadblocks— including a six-year-old and a crying toddler who would both insist on my staying home. That guilt, plus my general exhaustion, would probably prevail more often than not.

You've got to set yourself up to ensure that you have the least possible number of roadblocks. You won't be able to avoid them all every single day, but you have to try to the extent that it is practical. Occasionally, I forget my running clothes at home. Then I have a choice to make: take a day off if I have one available; listen to the screaming and pleas but go anyway; or take the kids with me. It's okay to have to make that choice once in a while, but making it every day would be painful and would easily kill my motivation. Instead, having workout clothes on and being ready to run as soon as I pull into the driveway (or at a trail before I even reach home) eliminates that scene altogether.

Many people who regularly work out feel like they have to do it in the morning or it won't get done. If you feel that way, and you have the motivation to get up early to do it, you should absolutely make morning your target time of day. Morning workouts are great for getting your body moving, strategizing about the day ahead, and giving yourself an overall sense of positivity going into the day. Truthfully, if I weren't so lazy (and possibly angry) in the morning, I'd like to experience the morning workout feelings. If I could show up to work with a better attitude, it'd be a more delightful scene for all.

If you choose to make morning your target time of day, you must know that if you hit the snooze button one too many times to get in your workout early, you have to make it up at some point during the day or evening. The target time of day isn't all or nothing. You have to be flexible in your approach. The end game is getting the workout in—whenever that may be—because that is another day that your streak remains alive. Working out is non-negotiable; the time you do it is always negotiable.

Some people who work outside the home choose the lunch hour to work out. If you can figure out the shower situation, this isn't a bad plan. Do you work from home? If you work at an office, is there a gym with a shower at the office? If the answer to either of these questions is yes, or if you don't mind stinking up the joint for half of each day, then a lunchtime workout might be for you.

Think about it—what do you really do during the lunch hour that is actually productive? If you could spend fifteen to thirty minutes of lunchtime briskly walking or running, then take a quick shower, you'd still have ten to fifteen minutes to eat. You could turn otherwise dead time into a productive activity. Plus, you could experience all the great feelings from a workout that can motivate you to get through the rest of the day. Going for a walk outside during the day always makes me feel better—if you do it regularly, you get that benefit daily and you keep the streak alive when you otherwise would be sitting around on social media or buying something online.

What if you get through the entire day and evening without working out, you've bathed the kids and put them to bed, and you just want to rest even though it is a critical streak day? You get your behind moving. "But I can't leave the kids here sleeping to go out and run!" You run inside, round and round and round until you hit your minimum. It's something you have to do. Get it done. It might be painful in the moment, but you will feel a thousand times better when your head hits that pillow knowing that you've kept your promise to yourself for one more day. Trust me. More importantly, that one more day means your streak and your motivation live on.

Great news. We've now discussed all the parameters you need to initially set up for endless streak success. But what about maintaining your streak long term? The following section will dive into the importance of recording your progress, planning for the week ahead, sacrificing when necessary to keep the streak alive, and addressing setbacks and injuries.

PART THREE:

MAINTAINING THE STREAK

8 RECORD YOUR PROGRESS

In any activity, a visual record of progress is exciting and fun. Pregnancy apps show you how big your baby is each week by comparing it to a fruit visual. "The baby is a kiwi this week!" you proudly declare to friends and family. If you have kids, you might have pen marks in the garage with dates next to them that show you and the kid how much growth progress is being made over time. If you are working on a financial goal, you might log into your bank account often to see the numbers—even though you generally know what they are—because seeing them in black and white makes progress feel even more real and exciting.

Just as well, keeping track of your progress with any activity keeps an accurate and simultaneous record so that you don't have to try to remember whether you did something or not. Think of crossing off items on a to-do list; maintaining an inventory of items; or marking emails as "unread" until you actually respond, then switching the status to "read" when you don't need to pay them any more attention.

Recording your streak progress is essential because it gives you a visual that will serve as further motivation. The record will also help you keep track to ensure that you don't miss an intended day, whether on purpose or by accident.

There are all sorts of methods you can use to record your progress. I like to record mine in the same planner I use for all my life organization purposes. I use a simple tick-mark system to keep track of my weekly five-day requirement. When I run more than three miles, I record that fact, as well as noting the mileage, because I like to know how often I'm running more significant distances. Admittedly, I'm not the best historian on the details of each workout, but I write down enough to see my progress and to ensure that I am truly doing five days per week.

You can do as little as I do or be more detailed in your approach. My boss's workout calendar looks like the most organized treasure map I've ever seen. It has symbols and lists and colors and even a key in case he forgets what it all means. He likes to record every imaginable detail so he can compare day to day, week to week, month to month, and year to year. He sets goals based on his history and progress. He ensures he's getting the desired variety by recording the type of exercise each day.

To me, that much recording would feel too heavy—like work. I think about exercise in a much simpler manner. Still, I do feel the need to make some record of what I'm doing, and when I take the time to look back and compare, I often surprise myself. "How did I train for a half marathon when I was that busy?" But these types of questions are often motivating—if I did it before through all the chaos, I can do it again.

Although I prefer old-fashioned manual recording, there are also plenty of apps to help with this sort of thing if you are more of a techie. Some will record your activities without you having to do anything except the exercise itself. These apps are particularly useful for ensuring you really did work out for your intended number of days.

The downside of using one of these apps comes if you want to take a good look at your history for any reason. Depending on how the information is stored, you may or may not be able to get a real grasp on your historical performance and how it compares to the present. And if you aren't recording the information together with whatever else is going on in your life (easier to do with a planner or on a calendar with all your other activities), it can be hard to remember life circumstances when reviewing your progress. This could be a missed opportunity to feel proud of yourself: "Wow, I still ran five days a week last December even with attending sixteen holiday parties!"

However you choose to do it, recording your streak progression is important, especially in the early phases. This will be a new experience. With each day that passes, you will see progress, whether it is in the time it takes you to run or walk or bike your intended mileage, or whether it is your ability to continue past the minimum, or whether it is the simple idea that you have continued exercising after not finding the motivation to do that prior to starting the streak. Showing yourself the progress will at least motivate you to keep going, and the possibilities beyond that motivation are endless.

Other than making a record, an unofficial way to "record" your progress is to tell your friends and family about it. Again, you know that I have not been great about this in the past. I can tell you, though, that it is very motivating for the few people who know or care about my streak to ask me about it. By now, it's such a part of the fabric of my being that people who are close to me occasionally ask, "Is the streak still alive?" The sort of rhetorical question they probably ask just for the hell of it. But after a major life event like a childbirth, people have asked the question surely expecting a negative response, only to be met with, "Sure is."

There is something oddly satisfying about surprising people who are skeptical of your ability to keep a streak intact. Also, if you are in the early stages of yours, telling your friends and family will serve as motivation because you won't want to go back on your word that you're starting a streak. All those skeptics will be waiting for you to fail at it—how satisfying will it feel to prove them wrong? Much more satisfying than having to admit during the next family dinner that you are no longer on the latest fad diet or workout program. Trust me.

In addition to (or instead of) telling your close friends and family about your streak progress, what about posting your progress on social media? Telling your followers about your progress will surely give you even more motivation not to quit.

Also, please tell me about it! You can find me through my publishing website, thewoodshoppellc.com (Contact tab), or on Instagram @ThePoweroftheStreak and Twitter @PowerofStreak. Also, you can hashtag your photos with #thepowerofthestreak. I want to hear if you've committed to starting a streak, and I want to hear about reaching particular milestones or goals. It's always fun to find like-minded people who are going through similar journeys. Follow me for streak inspiration, ideas, and maybe a laugh or two.

9 PLAN FOR THE WEEK AHEAD

Another essential step in maintaining your streak is to plan for the week ahead. This isn't an overly involved process but taking a few minutes to do it at the beginning of each streak week ensures that you get all of your days under your belt regardless of your life circumstances. Planning for the week may be the single most important factor in maintaining your streak.

You have to eliminate your weekly obstacles to the extent possible. Sure, there may be surprises, but for the most part, you'll be able to anticipate the obstacles and craft a plan to overcome them. Without anticipating and planning around your obstacles, they will feel impossible to overcome on a day-to-day basis. Before you know it, maintaining the streak will feel like too much work and you'll give up. You must set yourself up to avoid this feeling, to make it feel as easy as possible to get the workouts done.

I plan for the week by glancing at my weekly calendar on Monday, the day my streak week starts. Knowing I like to run at night and that I can take two days off, I check for any planned night activity that will make it really difficult to get a run in. This can be going to dinner with a friend right after work (I prefer not to show up reeking and sweaty although in truth, I will if necessary), a night meeting where I'll need to look presentable, a soccer practice for the six-year-old, or some other special occasion that will make running difficult.

Usually it breaks out to having one to two of these types of evenings per week, not including the weekends when I have more flexibility with the timing of the run. I don't like to start a weekend having to run both of the weekend days, so if I have two challenging nights during the week, I negotiate with myself. If it's soccer practice when I usually bring the one-year-old along in his stroller, I tell myself, "Running in the grass won't be that bad as long as I remember to put the nicer stroller in the car that morning." If it's dinner with my best pal, I think, "Maybe she won't mind meeting me at seven instead of six so I can run and shower beforehand." If it's a meeting, "I can run afterwards." Notice here that I'm not giving up the things I want or need to do. I'm simply finding a way to run around them.

Knowing the obstacles on the front end is important for setting expectations and planning. If I've committed to running after the meeting, I know I have to lace up as soon as I get home instead of having dinner and resting like I would otherwise do. If I'm going to try to convince my pal to meet me at seven in exchange for her not feeling sick during dinner by having to look at and smell me, I can reach out early in the week to allow her to plan in advance.

On the relatively rare occasions when I have so much going on that I just can't figure out how to get three or four runs in during the week at night, I know I have to make a serious sacrifice and get it done in the morning once or twice. Again, planning ahead is crucial.

Some weeks, I manage to run at night all five weekdays. Those occasions are extremely rare these days, but if I pull it off, I can rest the entire weekend guilt-free.

Your plan will be unique to you and will depend on a number of factors, including your amount of free time, your chosen number of days per week, your preferred workout time, and your overall life circumstance. What is important is that you have a plan and that you are willing to change it if need be in the name of keeping the streak alive.

If a random extra soccer practice pops up during the week and you have the joy of bringing the one-year-old as a special guest, you have to trudge through the grass with the stroller. If you forget the good stroller, well, good luck. Either you resolve to use the crappy one this time or figure out how to exercise after you get home. But get it done.

10 SACRIFICE WHEN NECESSARY

Another key to ensuring the livelihood of your streak is to sacrifice when necessary. This shouldn't be often if you are planning ahead and anticipating obstacles, but you will find that a rare occasion dictates sacrifice or serious streak jeopardy. I'm talking here about pivotal moments: situations you find yourself in that you can't necessarily anticipate, or even if you anticipate them, you wonder how you might be able to overcome them. Sometimes, you may even need a little luck on your side.

The biggest "sacrifice when necessary" moments for me came with pregnancy and childbirth. When I became pregnant with my first child, I had been maintaining my running streak for about five years. Of course when I started the streak, I had no thoughts whatsoever about becoming pregnant and certainly wasn't thinking about how I might handle any pregnancy down the road.

I remember vividly the first doctor appointment post-positive pregnancy test. My husband, nervous about the running and equally nervous about pissing me off, cautiously asked the doctor his thoughts about keeping my running streak alive. I, frankly, had no intention of asking. I had done enough googling to be satisfied that if running was already a part of my normal routine, I could safely do it during pregnancy.

The doctor looked confused. "What do you mean by 'running streak?'" Tyler then went on to explain to him that I run five days per week every single week, and I am religious about it. The doctor launched into a surely-canned speech about overdoing it and listening to your body. He reluctantly agreed that I could keep running regularly, as long as I promised to listen to my body and stop if my body told me to stop. Done.

And so, I ran. The first trimester wasn't bad. The second trimester wasn't good. The third trimester was hell. Like running with an eight-pound bowling ball in your tummy. Again, I told myself, "You can do anything for ten minutes," although the reality by bowling-ball status was probably twelve to fourteen. I'm not sure I made it past one mile on the dot during the entire third trimester.

I hate to admit it, but as the prospect of childbirth neared, I found myself worrying over whether the streak would end when the baby was born. Not because of some sick obsession that prioritized the streak over the birth of my first child, but because I had a fear that if the streak ended, I would never again get off the couch to go for another run. And this would happen at a time in my life when I could use exercise the most, both physically and mentally. Probably an irrational fear, but a real one.

For three weeks leading to the birth of my first child, I had terrible bouts of night contractions that would keep me up at all hours. They'd get intense, less than five minutes apart, I'd wake my husband and tell him to get ready for the hospital, and they'd fizzle out before we left. Over and over. During this period, my fears turned from my streak ending to accidentally having my baby at my house because of being faked out one too many times.

One Friday, two days before my due date, I was desperate to have the baby. I had reached that point— I imagine most mothers can relate—when the baby simply was no longer welcome in my stomach. Having failed at all other wives' tales/home remedies for ridding yourself of a full-term baby, I turned to running. The same me who could barely eke out one mile for the previous three plus months somehow managed to run more than four miles that morning. "There," I thought. "That'll do it."

That run did indeed jump-start contractions which, together with the help of some labor inducing drugs, resulted in the birth of my baby girl shortly before midnight. That cold Friday in February will go down as one of the best days of my life, despite trying to kill myself by running way more than I should have. I later paid for that run in awful pain that could have been worse than the typical post-childbirth stuff!

As the weekend drew to a close and we brought our darling baby girl home from the hospital, it occurred to me at one point that because I had run all five weekdays, my streak was still intact. And I could take off the entire weekend, plus the first two days of the following week to rest since my streak week started on Monday. Hmmm…

I decided not to think about it again until Wednesday, when the decision would have to be made to give it a go or kiss the streak goodbye. When Wednesday came, I wasn't feeling great but I thought I could physically do it. So why not give it a go?

I hate to know what the neighbors might have thought if they happened to glance out the window that day and saw a hunched, limping, spit-up-soaked woman attempting to run in a forward manner but more so appearing to be going backwards. I also would hate to google what actually qualifies as "running/jogging" and compare it to whatever poor attempt I engaged in that day. But you know what? I did it. I meaningfully attempted to run for one mile. Good enough in my book. The streak lived on.

For me, this was certainly a pivotal moment. I had a choice to make: let the streak die for a damn good reason or keep the streak alive. A little luck was required as well. I don't think there's any possible way I could have done that only one- or two-days post-childbirth. For whatever reason, the stars aligned in such a way that I was given the gift of four recovery days before deciding whether to attempt a run. Best not to waste that gift.

My doctor would tell you otherwise, and from a medical standpoint, he very well could be right. I'm certainly not urging you to ignore medical advice in pivotal moments. In fact, I'm convinced that my running so soon after my first born (and/or the infamous Friday four-miler just before the birth) is responsible for a lingering upper leg pain I still get six years later during longer runs. But for me, it was the right choice because I knew in my "heart of hearts" that I could do it, and I also knew that if I chose not to do it, I'd be breaking the streak promise to myself I made all those years earlier.

Plus, keeping the streak alive post-childbirth was critical to helping my body get back to its new normal (never the same, but close enough), and to mentally helping me get through those first few months. The short break and fresh air each day were welcome and needed. I also got a burst of energy with each run. All in all, the benefits of keeping the streak alive during that time far outweigh the leg pain I live with now.

As luck would have it, my second child, a boy weighing in at a perfect five pounds, was born on a Sunday after I completed all streak week requirements. The recovery with him was much easier, and by Wednesday I felt ready to give it a very gentle go. So, once again, a little luck and a lot of dedication resulted in the streak staying alive.

Pivotal moments come in all forms. My husband's most pivotal moment to date was several years ago during a cruise to the Bahamas. He had convinced himself going into the vacation that he'd have to end the streak because the pools on the ship would be too crowded and too small for him to swim his required laps in any meaningful way. Although the cruise was relatively short, there was simply no way for him to get in the required five days that week—any way he sliced it, he'd be short one. At that point, he was relatively early in his streak journey, and he was fine with this reality: he prioritized family time and a fun vacation over keeping the streak alive.

We took the vacation, did all the things, and found ourselves at the beautiful Atlantis resort to swim with dolphins. A must, obviously. After a lovely time in the dolphin pool—no, he did not count his time with the dolphins as his required lap swimming—we were walking back to our "base" area that we had set up near a water park full of slides and such. Out of the blue, right there in front of him, appeared a huge lap pool that was completely empty. Not a soul was around. Who'd swim laps at a place like that?

I actually saw Tyler's face light up in this pivotal moment. He had been given a gift and just happened to be dressed for the occasion. He was not going to waste this opportunity.

That one more day was all he needed to keep his swimming streak alive. So, the streak lived on through the vacation that he thought would make swimming laps impossible.

Another pivotal moment for Tyler came when the COVID-19 pandemic hit America. In March 2020, all gyms in our area closed, making it impossible for him to swim his laps. But then he realized: our local tennis club has outdoor pools. He decided to give it a go and see if they'd let him swim his laps. They agreed. But there was a problem. It was March and none of the pools were heated. Amazingly, he had enough dedication to swim in cool temperatures (thank goodness for Florida weather) with freezing water for three plus months, all in the name of keeping the streak alive.

If you do it long enough, there will be moments here and there that are pivotal. Moments in which you have a decision to make. Maybe you won't find yourself so lucky as to have a lap pool drop out of the sky when you need it, but if you do, you've got to seize the opportunity.

Aside from these types of situations that don't happen often, there are more regular occasions when you'll have to sacrifice to keep the streak alive. For instance, most of us (especially those with children) find ourselves sick with varying degrees of illness multiple times per year. Unless the illness is so severe that you physically can't do your streak activity, you have to buck up and get it done. It's surprising how much you can do—even when feeling terrible—if you put your mind to it. Besides, by now you should know what's coming next: you can do anything for ten minutes.

The key takeaway is that if you set up your streak the right way in the beginning and you take all steps to properly maintain it, sacrifice won't often be necessary. It'll be the rare exception rather than the rule. On those rare occasions when sacrifice becomes necessary, however, you've got to do it in the name of the streak.

11 SETBACKS AND INJURIES

You've done everything you can to set yourself up for success. You've sacrificed when able and necessary. You've kept the streak going for long enough to make it gel into part of your overall lifestyle. So what happens when you have a setback or injury that truly forces it to end?

The most important thing to remember if this happens is that all streaks end sooner or later. If you've really done all you can to keep your streak alive and circumstances outside of your control end it, you should look back on your streak with pride. But you should also look forward to starting again when you're able.

On the injury front, if you're doing any sort of physical activity, injury is inevitable. The question is whether the injury is so severe that you can't push through it. Only you know whether it's possible given your particular situation.

I've kept the streak going through shin splints, pesky knee twitches, and other minor injuries that have popped up here and there. Because my definition of a streak involves a relatively minor amount of physical exercise at a time, I've been able to push through injury with relative ease.

Early in my streak, I had a harsh incident when running with my Great Dane, Woodrow. He sensed we were close to home and started pulling hard on the leash. I sped up to keep up with him (never a good move), but I didn't realize the sidewalk was completely uneven from mature tree roots. I tripped over a crack in the sidewalk and flew through the air like Superman, still attached to the leash with the running dog. I finally landed on my side. It must have been quite a scene because a random stranger came to my aid.

Lucky for me, the worst bruise was to my ego, but I would later learn that I had relatively significant nerve damage on the landing side. This has caused me some pain, especially in my shoulder, but I work through it.

Other runners deal with pesky and painful sciatica issues while running. I feel for them because, having felt that nerve pain from time to time over the years, I know it is no fun. They get through it, though, because they've learned from a mental and physical standpoint to deal with the pain and push through it.

My friend Megan and I have both kept our streaks alive through minor surgical procedures. I still remember the infamous story about how she ran the morning of her surgery so that she'd have two recovery days afterwards (she's a five-dayer also). When the nurse attempted to put in her intravenous (IV) line, she had a hard time because Megan was slightly dehydrated from running just an hour earlier.

This sort of dedication will be crucial especially in moments of weakness when you are having physical pain or other emotional issues that make you not want to exercise.

If you falter, though, you can't give up.

First, you need to ask yourself why you faltered in the first instance. Was it because you tried everything you could but circumstances beyond your control just made it such that you temporarily couldn't continue? This type of scenario should be easy to overcome despite my illogical fear of the contrary with childbirth.

What about a time when you know you can push through but you choose not to? I think it's important to ask yourself why you made that choice.

Tyler found himself making a critical streak-day decision on the Sunday after our second child was born. I was still in the hospital, still an emotional mess, and still trying to figure things out with a newborn. He made the conscious decision, without discussing it with me, that it was more important to be with the baby and me in the hospital than to swim, even though it was the needed last day of his week. Had I known this to be the case that day, I would have insisted otherwise. That he chose to forego the streak day in favor of being there for those initial critical hours says a lot about his priorities.

But you know what? He gave himself a mulligan that day. He knew and could be honest with himself that his decision did not come down to laziness or lethargy or not caring. Instead, he cared more deeply about being there for that important life moment. Although I haven't personally been faced with the prospect of having to take a mulligan, I like the idea. It has to be reserved for those big life moments though. Not because the latest Netflix special came out and you have to binge.

If your streak ends and you reflect and realize that you could have worked out but chose not to for a reason that wasn't very important, then maybe you should reevaluate the streak entirely. Start by re-reading this book. Then ask yourself: do you need to redefine the streak? Either by changing the minimum days per week, amount of exercise, or even the type?

My boss, who has the longest and most impressive workout streak of anyone I know, had an original six-month streak end years ago when he was traveling often. One particular day, he found himself in an airport with an unexpected layover, meaning that he simply wouldn't be able to get in his required thirty minutes of cardio. So, his streak was over.

When he reflected on his lifestyle at the time that included heavy traveling, he decided he needed to redefine his streak requirements to include brisk walking. This would still count as cardio and would allow him to get in his required thirty minutes no matter what because he can walk anywhere—even in an airport.

The result of this self-reflection and a small tweak in requirements has been more than seventeen years of the new streak staying alive and well.

Whatever the reason for your streak ending, a little self-reflection will go a long way in starting a new one. And when you start a new one, make your first goal to outlast your initial streak. This will give you some needed motivation to really jump start it again and keep it going. Then, when you meet that goal, you'll feel accomplished and want to keep going.

Any injury or setback can be overcome. You just need to reflect on what caused it in the first instance, and whether, moving forward, you need to change some things.

PART FOUR:

BEYOND THE STREAK

12 SET OTHER FITNESS GOALS TO ACHIEVE WHILE KEEPING UP YOUR STREAK

By now you know that the streak is so powerful because it ensures you keep working out through any chaos life may throw at you. But what if you are not getting your desired result in terms of overall fitness, or if you just have the urge to do more than the minimum? Simple. You set higher workout goals to achieve. You guessed it, though, you have to keep the streak alive through these other goals.

Maybe I've convinced you that a one-mile run is the way to go for your streak activity. Great! Get started today!

What you'll notice over time is that having the streak will change the way you view yourself. There is a certain level of confidence you'll have just by keeping the streak alive. This will start spilling over into other areas, like healthy eating and other habits. Remember, this is a cynic talking—if I would have been told ten years ago that I'd actually develop an aversion to chocolate and sweets, I would have spit out my drink and scoffed. With time, though, you begin to realize the actual, practical benefits of fitness. Whether consciously or subconsciously, those benefits spill over into other areas. A compound effect starts. Before you know it, you'll want to do more. Trust me.

If you reach a point where you want to do more than the minimum streak exercise, there are countless ways to achieve it. First, you could sign up for and train for an organized run. As I've mentioned, I've participated in several handfuls of these over the years. They typically vary in distance from 5k (3.1 miles) to 10k (6.2 miles) to 15k (9.3 miles), all the way to a half marathon (13.1 miles) and a full marathon (26.2 miles). Sometimes there are one milers. And for those who are hopeless gluttons for punishment, there are even ultramarathons (anything longer than a standard marathon).

Some people choose one or two organized runs or events per year and sign up for them every time, without fail. This method could be like a streak within your streak! Plus doing one or two organized runs or events per year will ensure that you train at least every six months or year beyond your minimum requirements.

My city holds an annual River Run 15k, and there are handfuls of runners who have run every single time since its inception in 1978. They're affectionately referred to as the "streakers," and they even get this designation on their race numbers. How cool is that?

Within about two months of starting my own running streak, I participated in my first 5k organized run. At the time, my boss convinced me that it was a good idea to have a little more motivation to keep the streak alive in those early days. It did serve to motivate me, and I'm glad I did it. Running that 5k was the most I had ever run in my life at the time. I felt a sense of accomplishment way beyond the two-month streak I then had going.

What I've learned over the years is that if an organized run is too crowded or chaotic, it simply isn't for me. I have a hard enough time with anxiety as it is. I don't need to be worried about tripping over people who decide on a dime to walk for a minute, or drunken spectators throwing mini donut holes to runners. So, if I do participate in organized runs these days, I look for smaller, less popular runs. Sure, I still have to deal with being left in the dust by women pushing strollers (seriously?!), but I can handle the overall environment a lot better if I have a little space.

Other people thrive on the energy and organized chaos of popular runs. Plus, the popular ones always have the most fun post-race parties. Yes, there are parties, sometimes with free beer. You even get a medal and a t-shirt most of the time. These things in and of themselves are motivation for finishing.

My husband, Tyler, has run a few 5ks, several River Runs in a row, and even a half marathon since starting his swimming streak (he sucked up the back pain temporarily to the extent he could). Being in better physical shape from swimming has allowed him to complete these runs when he otherwise would struggle mightily.

My boss, who may or may not be human, has run a marathon, countless half marathons, has done at least two organized 100-mile bike rides (one in the Rockies), and sets truly incredible periodic fitness goals for himself that he almost always achieves.

I recommend trying an organized event, especially if you haven't done one before. Trust me, you'll see people from all walks of life. There is no shame, only encouragement. Whether it be an organized run, bike race, triathlon, swimming event, or something else entirely, the sheer act of signing up for the event a couple of months in advance will provide you with motivation to do more than your minimum streak requirements. No matter what type of activity you choose to sign up for, there are countless training guides out there to ensure you are ready for the big day. Just google your type of event (i.e. "5k run") and "training guide."

If organized runs/races/events aren't for you (I get it), there are so many other ways to motivate yourself beyond the minimum of the streak. If you're running or walking, you could set a goal of a certain number of miles per week, or of achieving a specific number in a month. Just don't overdo it—you want to avoid injury.

When I'm working up to something other than my minimum of one mile, I start by increasing just two or three of my weekly runs to about two miles. Then, the second week, I keep two runs at two miles, and aim for at least three miles with one run. The third week, I may do one run for two miles, two runs for three miles, and a single run for four miles.

You want to gradually build a base of miles so that your body isn't shocked by all the extra. The same can be said for any other type of physical activity: elliptical, walking, biking, swimming, etc. Again, there are lots of great training manuals and blogs out there for building up to a certain number of miles or laps.

If you want to do something more than your minimum, how about trying another exercise entirely?

This will give you some variety and allow you to experiment. I've tried biking, dancing, swimming, yoga, weight training, and core work to name a few, all while keeping my running streak alive. My next experiment will be kickboxing as it sounds like fun! Because my streak has such a low minimum requirement, taking on other activities, especially for a defined period of time, is not that much of a strain.

Currently, in my attempt to achieve pre-baby physique (a seemingly impossible feat the second time around), I have a goal to do core work three times per week. Sometimes I meet it; sometimes I don't. This says a lot about the Power of the Streak. I know I *have to* run. At the same time, while I really don't want to have a flabby stomach anymore, I only have the motivation to do what I need to do on that front *sometimes*. Why? I don't have a core work streak. I have a running streak. Nevertheless, I continue to set the core goal in the hope that I'll achieve it.

It's important not to redefine your streak requirements just because you get excited about doing more than the minimum. Remember, we are focused on longevity for the streak. If I were to add a requirement of doing core work three times per week to the streak requirement, that would add thirty or so minutes to my workout routine three times per week indefinitely. That is not sustainable for my lifestyle in the long term. So, while it is great to set goals within your streak, be careful not to get too excited about your extra motivation and redefine the streak to include exercise that is not going to be sustainable.

At the same time, if you have worked hard doing your streak exercise and know you are ready for more, as long as you are thoughtful about it and adequately consider the long-term effects, it may be appropriate to reevaluate your minimum. Maybe you started walking but are now confident you can run. Maybe you started with half a mile but are now confident you can do one mile. These sorts of logical progressions are good, as long as you're thinking them through.

Back to goals beyond your streak minimum, any goal is great. Sometimes I have the motivation to achieve the goal; sometimes I don't even try. That's the beauty of the set up though. I know I have a baseline of fitness throughout my life, regardless of whether I have motivation. When I feel particularly motivated, I try for another goal. But even if I don't achieve it, I have the streak to fall back on.

While writing this book, I got so inspired that I started training for a half marathon. Ultimately, I decided not to go forward for a lot of reasons, including the time of year and the sheer time dedication involved in writing while simultaneously training. So, I made the decision to pull the plug on it for now. I think I'll try again when things don't feel quite so hectic. This is the first time I have started training for an organized run and decided not to do it. While the decision does feel a bit deflating, I'm good with it because I know I'll try again sometime soon. And of course I know I'll keep running.

Amazingly though, my "long run" mileage plunged from a ten-miler just a couple short weeks ago, to currently about three miles. I've temporarily lost motivation for distance running without a goal looming, but because of my streak, I won't lose motivation for running altogether. That's an important distinction to remember, even if you don't meet your goals.

Fitness goals beyond the minimum of your streak are fun and give you additional motivation. Plus, you can be creative in what you choose to try and how often you try it, knowing you will always have your streak to fall back on, even if you don't meet your other goals.

13 STREAKING IN AREAS OTHER THAN FITNESS

The streak concept is particularly powerful if you really buy in. I think it works best in the exercise area of life because that is an area that feels so hard to stay motivated. But the streak mentality can also work well in other areas of life, especially if you are trying to meet a longer-term goal.

Ever tried to learn a foreign language? Achieve a goal of reading a certain number of books per year? Saved for a big purchase? These are all areas that are ripe for applying the streak concept, but an important distinction between these areas and fitness is that your fitness streak should remain alive indefinitely. Streaks in other life areas are difficult to maintain indefinitely and should be started with the idea in mind that there is a logical "end goal."

I currently have a streak of practicing Italian on my favorite app for more than 1,000 nights in a row. I started learning the language thinking we were taking a trip to Italy. Thanks to a global pandemic, the trip got cancelled—twice—but for some reason I have kept the streak alive for about three years now despite no trip in immediate sight. I can't exactly describe why because I'm not even remotely close to fluency at this point. I basically do the one-lesson minimum just to say I did it. There is something about the streak concept and the longevity I've already built up that makes me not want to stop. Plus, maybe someday I'll finally get to go to Italy and can attempt to order my coffee or pasta like a local.

The streak concept also works well to help you achieve a longer-term goal outside of exercise because it allows you to break the goal down into smaller, more actionable steps. For instance, say you have a goal of reading twenty books next year. If the average book is 200 pages, you'll need to read 4,000 total pages. If you commit to reading each night, you know you'll need to average just under eleven pages per night to reach your goal. Wow! That's not much at all. If you commit to the nightly reading streak, you'll easily meet your goal by the end of the year.

The same idea can apply to achieving a financial goal. Maybe you decide your goal is to save $10,000 in a year. That's roughly $833 per month. What streak can you implement for the year that will allow you to achieve that monthly goal? Remember, this is a longer-term concept. Resigning yourself to "not eating out" for an entire year is probably not going to get you very far. But what if you took on a side job for a year? Something that would earn you a little more than $200 weekly. This essentially amounts to a streak of working a certain number of extra hours per week for a defined period of time. This is sustainable over a longer term and would allow you to achieve your greater goal.

These are just a couple of examples of how the streak concept can apply to other areas of life. While I do endorse the streak concept in some non-fitness areas of life, I caution you to not let the concept overtake you. It really can be effective in helping you achieve goals, but life is not easily broken into rigid categories. For me, the most important streak—the one not to be broken—is the exercise streak because it is sustainable indefinitely and because fitness is so important to overall health.

14 INSPIRING OTHERS THROUGH YOUR FITNESS STREAK

The last—and potentially most exciting—exercise streak concept we should explore is how you can inspire others with your streak. Face it, we all know handfuls of people who can use some regular exercise. How can we help them achieve it without being pushy or preachy?

Until now, I've admittedly not done a great job with being intentional about inspiring others. Despite my failings, I have unintentionally inspired several people close to me to start their own streaks just by the sheer act of keeping my streak alive. You've read the stories of my husband and my friends. When people see you doing something seemingly difficult and doing it consistently, no matter what the circumstance, it is inspiring in and of itself. They associate you with doing something out of the ordinary; something that sets you apart.

Even if people don't realize I have a running streak, they often come to me for advice or encouragement when they start working out. Why? Because I'm often seen in workout clothes, and I'm often seen out running. Whether it's at the coffee shop, the playground, daycare, or anywhere else, people tend to associate me with fitness just because I dress the part (and sometimes smell it too). Plus, I am told countless times per year by various people in my professional and personal lives, "I saw you running the other day!"

For years and years, I had no real desire to inspire others when it came to fitness. It was just something I did for myself. But as I age and I see what life does to us middle-agers and beyond, I become more and more interested in finding ways to help others achieve fitness goals. We should all have a level of interest in this concept. Caring about others means caring about their physical health.

As I mentioned in the beginning, one of the ways I'm choosing to inspire others is through writing this book. I'm in the game of hoping that it helps people who are struggling with a consistent workout routine like I once was. I'm also choosing to donate a portion of the royalties to a charitable cause that is near to my heart and helps others with staying fit.

Another way I'm inspiring others is by teaching my children the benefits of running. I'm proud to say my six-year-old can consistently run a mile, and I'm even more proud to report that she just completed her very first 5k. These are things I never dreamed of doing at her age.

When you start your own streak, how will you inspire others? How will you pay it forward in your own way?

I'm so excited for you—you've made it to the end of this book, so I know you have the motivation to do it. Now get out there and get it done! And please, come tell me about starting your streak or ask any questions you may have. I'm on Instagram @ThePoweroftheStreak, on Twitter @PowerofStreak, or you can find me through my publishing website: thewoodshoppellc.com. Good luck to you!

ABOUT THE AUTHOR

Kara Wood lives in a suburb in Florida. She's an ordinary person, the opposite of a fitness expert. What is perhaps extraordinary about Ms. Wood, however, is her ability to keep a running streak alive for twelve years and counting—through a challenging career as an attorney; two pregnancies and childbirths; being a wife and mother; and all of the other challenges and chaos that life has thrown her way.

Write to Ms. Wood at mail@thewoodshoppellc.com. She'd love to hear from you.

Authors published by The Wood Shoppe, LLC proudly donate twenty percent of all author royalties to a non-profit charitable cause of their choice. For more information about the charity benefitting from the purchase of this book, visit TheWoodShoppeLLC.com.

Printed in Great Britain
by Amazon

29481720R00070